This is me!

To Eva and Nina

As we pass life on

This is me!

Becoming who you are
using Transactional Analysis

Lieuwe Koopmans

Published by
Sherwood Publishing
Wildhill, Broadoak End, Hertford SG14 2JA, UK

www.sherwoodpublishing.com
email: sherwood@psychologicalintelligence.com

First published 2017
Version 2 Published 2019
First published in Dutch in 2012 by Thema, Zaltbommel, NL

A catalogue record of this book is available from the British Library.

ISBN 978-1-907037-08-5

Design by Diane Richardson, info@drdm.eu
Printed by CMP (UK) Ltd www.cmp-uk.com

This is me!

Become who you are with Transactional Analysis

We live in a society in which we think that happiness in life can be engineered. We watch programmes on T.V. about total makeovers and diets, about raising children and about financial problems. We hope the experts featuring on those programmes will solve our problems, in order for us to be happy. On YouTube and Facebook we reveal how special we are and the wonderful life we are having. Problems don't exist; everything is great and fantastic. And so we become actors of our own lives.

But what is left once you remove the wonderful stories and the outer shell? *This is me!* invites you to search for your true self. The book raises questions and gives practical examples and direction. To guide you on your way, Lieuwe Koopmans uses Transactional Analysis (TA), a theory of personality and model for communication combined. The accessible models and lines of thinking enable you to better understand complex psychological processes and they can also be used as tools for personal and professional growth. This is a unique book that will help you increase your self-knowledge and self-awareness.

This is me! let's you take a look at how your past affects your current behaviour. Considering that an important part of the answers to your life's questions are locked up in your own past, TA is a wonderful way to look at the various parts within yourself. You will gain insight into your own reality, your frame of reference. This is the basis upon which you will be able to increase your options for how to behave and to treat yourself and others in a respectful manner. With the help of TA you can become an autonomous human being who is able to live in the-here-and-now with love and awareness.

Lieuwe Koopmans

Foreword

It is a special pleasure for me to write this Foreword as the publisher as well as being a Transactional Analysis trainer with many years commitment to sharing TA with others. In addition to commenting here, therefore, on an important addition to the TA literature, I can share my enjoyment of the process of taking a successful book in Dutch and bringing it to a wider audience.

When I first read the early translations, I could see immediately that this book would be valuable to the TA community, and especially to our clients, students, families, friends and colleagues. Lieuwe has an accessible style of writing, draws on numerous examples in a way that brings the theory to life, and entertains the reader by using a format that mirrors a stage production, with a Prologue, five Acts and an Epilogue. He supplements this effectively with quotes from Shakespeare, reinforcing the perspective of us being players on the stage, which of course resonates with the Transactional Analysis ideas about operating within our own life script.

Lieuwe adds a range of significant TA concepts to supplement the readers' understanding of how they have created, and can therefore update, their own life stories. Readers are provided with several different models to enable them to increase self-awareness and identify new options for healthy functioning.

This is all 'topped' and 'tailed' with Chapters – Acts – that focus on the role of the vital energy for growth that Eric Berne referred to as physis, and to which Lieuwe adds thymos as passion and courage. Hence physis to grow and thymos for courage are what we need to take off our masks or make-up, and move beyond the limitations that we unknowingly adopted in childhood.

I am delighted, therefore, to have been involved in making this valuable material available. Whether you are new to Transactional Analysis or have, like me, spent years studying, applying and teaching it to others, you will find many nuggets of value within this book.

Julie Hay
Teaching & Supervising Transactional Analyst (Counselling, Organisational, Psychotherapy & Educational)

Contents

Acknowledgments

This book is the fruit of my own developmental journey over the past 50+ years.

I start with deep gratitude to all teachers I have had the privilege of meeting along this path. I am exceptionally grateful to Piet Weisfelt and Wibe Veenbaas. They were the ones who pointed the existence of this path out to me.

Sander Rainalda has been my study partner and very dear friend for over twenty years. During the process of writing this book, Sander watched over the purity of my TA-thinking. Very memorable are all our walks together during which he sharpened my thoughts.

Ton Lansdaal, a layperson in TA, gave up his time to read the texts I produced and to see whether outsiders would be able to comprehend what I had written.

Monique Lindzen, editor at Uitgeverij Thema, was possibly an even more critical outsider. Again and again she pushed me to make my text more accessible, even though it all seemed very logical to me in the first place. Her persistence has proved to be of greater service to the development of my writing skills than it has been for me to write this book.

I am also grateful to Thema's willing consent to publish this book in English.

Roek Lips was my sparring partner on several critical occasions during the writing process. Partly thanks to his ideas, I was able to get back on track.

Jos Vermij and I have been life partners for over thirty years. During this time, we have experienced the contents of this book together in real life. In the process of writing, Jos tirelessly and critically read all my texts, always prepared to engage in joined-up thinking.

I owe a great deal of thanks to Leona Bishop for the splendid and accurate translation of my book from Dutch into English. Being bilingual and also having an understanding of TA is quite special. I am grateful she crossed my path.

This brings me to Julie Hay, my English publisher and source of inspiration in TA. After reading the translation of the introduction and first chapter of the book, she was prepared to edit the final translated version and release it on the English-speaking market. I am exceptionally grateful to Julie for making my dream come true.

And finally, a deep gratitude to all the people with whom I have had the privilege to work with during the past thirty years. The stories they shared with me have been an inexhaustible source of inspiration for my thinking with regard to 'humanity'.

Lieuwe Koopmans
Lieuwe Koopmans works as a trainer, coach, counsellor and organisational consultant for both the non-profit- and profit sectors. He has his own company. Via this he offers a variety of trainings and courses in the field of Transactional Analysis in cooperation with others (www.lieuwe.net). Furthermore, he works internationally as a trainer for Functional Fluency (www.functionalfluency.com). Since writing this book, Lieuwe has become internationally endorsed as a TA trainer and supervisor (TSTA Organisational).

All the world's a stage,

And all the men and women merely players.

They have their exits and their entrances,

And one man in his time plays many parts.

– William Shakespeare, 'As You Like It', Act 2, Scene 7

Prologue

On the first day of the Leadership Development Program, Carl focuses on 'connecting and letting go'. That night, he sleeps uneasily. In his mind's eye, he replays the film of the day. Then he reaches a decision. In the opening round of the second day, he calls for attention and tells the group it's his son's birthday. He would have turned seven if he hadn't died two years ago. 'Today is an important day to me,' he concludes. The group regards him in silence, while he examines their faces one by one.

Caroline is a 35-year-old cheerful and outgoing woman whose initial questions concern her career. 'Ultimately, I'm never passionate about what I do,' she tells me. 'It's as if a job never really touches me.' She explains she is on the lookout for a job that will evoke this passion in her. During one of our follow-up meetings we discuss her family background. She smiles and tells me that the answers to her questions are not to be found there. 'It really was a wonderful family. My dad went to work and my mum took care of everything at home. We never had to do anything.' Without any prompting, she tells me that her mother always did their laundry, made their sandwiches and cleaned up their rooms. She also mentions that her father was always prepared to drive them to their sports club when it rained. She ends on a significant note: 'So...' I complete her sentence: 'So you never really needed to struggle.'

Christine is a manager in the building industry and has been attending the group for two months. She is a quiet, withdrawn woman, who rarely raises a question and only briefly responds to what others contribute. Today, the group leader addresses Christine and explicitly invites her to contribute a case. She does so. During the first fifteen minutes, it's slow going. As soon as the group leader and the other group members pointedly question the relevance of this case to her own history, Christine begins to stutter.

All of a sudden, she seems to have taken a decision. The words begin to flow: about her Jewish background and her parents' experiences in a concentration camp, about their silence about this during her childhood, how her mother died at a young age, how she went to live with foster parents when she was ten, because her father couldn't raise her alone. 'I've never told this to anyone besides my husband.' Another group member asks how it feels for her to share her story. She smiles and answers: 'It's not bad at all.' And after a brief silence she repeats: 'Not bad at all...'

Three people, each with their own history: one who suffered a loss, another with whom nothing appears to be the matter, and a third with a traumatic childhood. The three histories also have something important in common. In the course of their lives, all three adapted to their situation. They did so by denying aspects of their personal history and hiding these from the world and quite possibly from themselves as well. In doing so, they denied the relevance of their personal history to their current life. Due to this adaptation, none of them show their true face. Instead, they have become someone who is not authentic: a 'strong man', a 'withdrawn woman' or a 'lucky dog'. It's like they pulled a mask over their faces or as if they modified their faces more subtly with cosmetics to make themselves look slightly different from the person they really are.

As if they modified their own faces with cosmetics to make themselves look slightly different from the person they really are.

Then they modified their behaviour accordingly, as if they are playing a part in the theatre of their own life. This is an increasingly common occurrence in the modern world. We are in the process of designing a society where having a perfect life is the highest attainable goal. It encourages suppressing or whitewashing anything that isn't perfect.

Countless television programmes are conveying the message that happiness can be manufactured. They include elimination shows, total makeovers, including for your house, and talent shows for dancers and singers in which we participate in multitudes. You're a pathetic loser if you don't go through life as a success. So we fill our Facebook page with messages that display our happiness to the world. We travel far and wide, have special experiences and record them in pictures and videos to show how special they were after we've returned.

And so we turn into actors in our own lives.

This has some ugly side effects. Playing a part in your own life may cause great sadness and lead to miscommunication. And we even gloat over these side effects. Other people's misfortune can be the source of entertainment or *Schadenfreude*, as the Germans say: a secret rejoicing in other people's misery and failure, to confirm our own good luck. Once again, the media play an important role, with YouTube videos and TV shows that reinforce this notion of being entertained by the misfortunes of others.

If you hide or distort your own history, your personal development will come to a halt. You will develop cracks behind the facade you put up, which render your life story less coherent. The show you put up agrees less and less with how you feel inside.

Swiss psychologist Carl Jung distinguished between the 'perfect life' and the 'full life'. In the perfect life, some parts of your personality must be denied and repressed. There is no room for anxiety, sadness, anger or failure. The full life, on the other hand, accommodates and provides meaning to everything: sadness and joy, good and evil, enjoyment and boredom, success and failure.

As German philosopher Friedrich Nietzsche said: 'You must become who you are.' That is a wonderful statement in this context. What happens if you aspire to the full life? What happens if you wipe the makeup from your face and put aside the mask? What is the meaning of the naked face that is revealed? What is the value of your lines, wrinkles and furrows? What do they represent?

In the past thirty years I have worked as a psychiatric nurse, (interim) manager, organisational consultant, counsellor, coach and trainer. Time and again I was struck by the importance of the real life story and the need to tell it in full and give it new significance. Whether it concerns successful people who want to become more successful, or people dealing with personal issues, or whose career is in danger of being sidelined, an important part of the answer lies hidden in their own history. This history profoundly affects how we interact and communicate in our present surroundings.

You may find answers to your life questions through the process of un-covering. The answer is already there; you only need to pull away the cover. That may be painful, although sometimes surprisingly simple. In almost all cases it will lead to renewed significance and new energy. This book may serve as a guide to this process, a guide for explorers, so to speak.

This book is intended for people who yearn for the full life. Reading this book may help you to view your personal history and the ways in which it affects your current behaviour with fresh eyes. In this way, it helps you to attach new significance to aspects of your life). In this manner, it will help you deal with questions that concern you now. This book prompts questions, provides examples and gives you a sense of direction. But it is up to you to take the necessary steps yourself.

Over the past thirty years, I have thoroughly studied many schools of psychology. Of these, Transactional Analysis has had the most profound impact on me. Transactional Analysis (frequently called TA in this book) is both a theory of personality and a communication model. It studies people's developmental history and its impact on their communication styles. With its simple, accessible models and conceptual frameworks, TA provides insight into complex mental processes and gives a large variety of tools for personal and professional growth. Moreover, it frequently employs theatrical concepts and metaphors. For these reasons Transactional Analysis has been the main inspiration for the content, design and structure of this book.

This book will take you on the following journey.
Following this Prologue, the First Act will commence. It is called 'The Unspoilt Life' and deals with human development from early childhood. It is an idealisation that no human being will ever really experience.

The Second, Third and Fourth Acts deal with how we put on makeup or masks in order to play our parts in life, and how we interact with other people in this guise. In each act, I will suggest opportunities for removing the makeup or taking off the mask.

The Second Act is called 'Masks and Makeup: The Cosmetics of Life'. It describes how we learn to put on makeup in order to adjust to circumstances and to prepare ourselves for our role.

The Third Act, 'The Life Script', describes how we make life choices and develop something of a life plan.

The Fourth Act, 'How the Script Is Formed', delves more deeply into topics from the third act. It describes the mechanisms that lead to script formation and discusses strokes (units of recognition) and emotions.

The Fifth Act, 'The Pageant', describes how our life script affects the way we design relationships in the present.

The Epilogue is a brief discussion of the courage needed to turn your life around.

Finally, in the annexes you will find a list of books per chapter, articles and/or websites that inspired me, a bibliography as well as some background material about TA. I trust that my predecessors will be sufficiently honoured in this manner.

I occasionally deviate from my own setup. To improve the flow and comprehensibility of the story, I occasionally thought it wise to anticipate a topic that is discussed later on or to re-emphasise something discussed earlier. That's how it works with stories: they refuse to let themselves be trapped by a pre-formed plan, but find their own way.

The book includes many questions and assignments that may help you during your personal investigation. I have also provided many examples. All of these were inspired by meetings with real people. With the exception of the examples about myself, none of the examples can be directly attributed to a single person. The three cases from the prologue return under the heading 'Interlude'. I use these cases to illustrate topics discussed in the preceding chapters. I frequently provide pointers for development.

One last thing: forty years ago, my father, who was a minister, wrote a Christmas play about Agape. Agape was a little boy who lived in a country where everybody wore a mask. He decided he didn't want to wear one and buried his in the garden. By doing so, he invited others to follow his example and look at themselves as they truly were. The Sunday school teacher asked me to play the part of Agape and that is how I, as a nine-year-old, came to invite people to take off their mask, unaware at that time of the deeper significance of this.

This story was at the back of my mind while I wrote this introduction. It made me realise how strongly this book is rooted in my own history.

Lieuwe Koopmans

First Act:
The unspoilt life

1. Vital Energy

A merry heart goes all the day, your sad tires in a mile-a.

William Shakespeare, 'The Winter's Tale', Act 4, Scene 3

I am sitting by my window, peering over the courtyard of the building complex where I live. It's almost the end of March and spring is in the air. The buds are reappearing on the rhododendrons. The daffodils are in bloom. Birdcalls had woken me early in the morning. I hear neighbourhood children shouting from among the shrubs. They're building a hut together. They instruct each other as if they've been doing it for years. Upstairs, my eldest daughter is studying for her exams. My youngest daughter is away rehearsing for a play. And me, I'm about to embark on this book. In short, everything is in motion; everything is growing and developing as if it had been put into action by an invisible force.

Why are people so concerned with growth and development? Why does my neighbour go to Australia to start a new life? Why does a pianist study a difficult section of one of Beethoven's compositions with endless discipline? Why does a mathematician doggedly attempt to solve a complex calculation?

Why do you…?

Stop and think: what's driving you?

What do you want to achieve:
> **professionally?**
> **in your private life; with your family or friends?**
> **in your leisure time, hobbies or sports?**

Have you set any goals for yourself or do you harbour any secret desires?

In TA, the invisible force behind the continual growth is called 'physis'. This is one of TA's central concepts: people's capacity for growth. Physis means the change or growth that comes from the spirit within the person. It could be translated as 'vital energy'. The concept dates from Ancient Greece and was introduced by the philosopher Heraclites, who said: 'We descend and do not descend into the same river; we are and are not.' By this he meant that we are constantly changing and consequently are never the same. Everything changes and everything moves. Eric Berne, the founder of TA, coined the term 'physis' to denote people's inner drive towards wholeness and health. In TA, which frequently uses symbols and metaphors, physis is always represented as an arrow pointing straight upward. This arrow is called the aspiration arrow, the 'arrow of desire'.

The aspiration arrow

The concept of physis encompasses six drives that encourage us to grow:

The power to live is the core drive that every healthy person experiences in life.

The power to be free is closely connected to the power to live. It is the power on the basis of which people organise and design their lives. This is the power that helps people distance themselves from limiting circumstances – relationships, jobs and other straightjackets.

The power to have new experiences, both in your inner world and in the world outside. People are naturally curious and keen to investigate. This may take the form of travels to distant countries, a new job, bungee jumping or reading a great book.

The power to take decisions and set your own course. Even though we all need to deal with the authority of others, on essential issues we have a profound need to decide for ourselves who and what we are, and what we feel and do.

The power to enter into authentic relationships. Every human being longs for an open and personal connection with others. Humans are relational creatures.

The power to experience life's spiritual dimension and to rise above oneself. In our present life this may well be the most frequently denied power and therefore the one most difficult to experience. Spirituality revolves around the experience of self-transcendence. For one person this will involve being in touch with what he or she calls God, for another the profound relationship with another human being, and for yet another being in touch with nature.

These six drives generate your main life values. If you can give these values a name, they may help you to infuse your own life with shape and purpose.

Annette and I discuss the things she considers important in life. She mentions three main values: 'freedom', 'real connections' and 'space for personal growth'. I ask her to outline an aquarium on the flipchart, to draw three rocks in it and to write down the words in these rocks. After she's done, I ask her to think of some other values she also considers to be important, although less important than the first three. I ask her to draw these as smaller rocks between the big ones. Finally, I ask her to include values that she considers of minor importance. In the conversation that evolves, we discuss the fact that people tend to fill their lives with 'grains of sand' of unimportance, leaving no room for the 'rocks' that they consider genuinely meaningful.

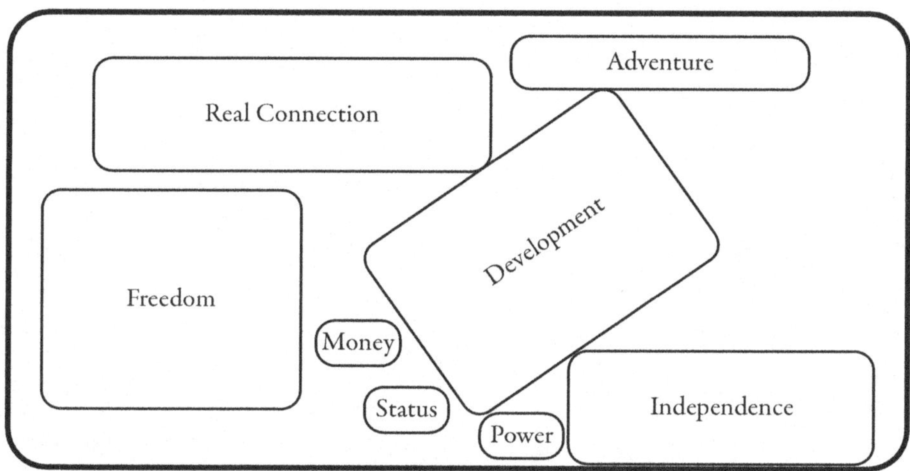

Annette's aquarium

This visualisation provides Annette with a perspective on the things in her life that she considers important. It enables her to let her choice of a new job coincide with her personal drives.

Assignment

> **Write down three values that you consider important in your life.**
> **Draw an 'aquarium' on a piece of paper, similar to the one described and shown above.**
> **Put your three big rocks inside and write down words that express the values.**
> **Add some smaller rocks, labelled with less important values.**

End with 'pebbles' that have less significance for you.
Consider whether the picture reflects the life you currently lead.
If the picture does not reflect the life you currently lead, consider how this affects your vital energy.
What can you/would you like to do differently?

2. Bonding and development

Love is not love when it is mingled with regards that stand aloof from the entire point.

William Shakespeare, 'King Lear', Act 1, Scene 1

In the previous chapter we started our journey with the concept of vital energy, the power that incites you to take action in your life. The foundation of your life energy, and the way you shape it, is laid down during the early years of your childhood. To gain insight on your own patterns of how you enter into relationships in the here-and-now, it is crucial to look back on the way you learnt to do this early in life.

In this chapter, I will discuss two important aspects related to the above: bonding and the cycles of development. I will give a description of how bonding and developing can evolve in an ideal way. Further on in the book I will give a comprehensive explanation of the less ideal paths one may take and how these paths lead us to wear 'makeup' or 'masks'.

Bonding
Attachment forms the foundation for a child's physical, cognitive and psychological development. It starts with a bond that develops between a child and his or her parents or primary caregiver, usually the mother. The forming of this bond in early childhood is necessary for the child to be able to connect with others later on in life.

In the bonding process, a number of steps can be distinguished, illustrated in the figure below and with an example:

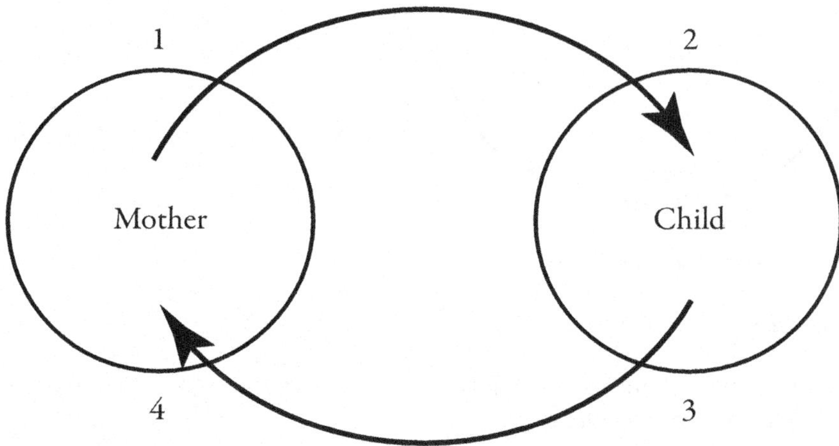

1.   The first step in the bonding process is the mother who connects with her child.
     Her child was so very welcome from the moment she knew she was pregnant.
     After giving birth, holding her child close, she felt warm gushes of love streaming through
     her body.

2.   The next step is up to the child wanting to receive
     When she lays her hand on the baby's stomach, she can feel that it soothes him and notices
     how he moves towards her hand. When he cries, she picks him up and cherishes him and
     it calms him down.

3.   The third step is up to the child, wanting to reach out to the mother.
     Lying in his cradle, he stretches his arms out to her and laughs.

4.   The last step is up to the mother, able to receive.
     She feels so close to him when he's holding on to her, as if he will never let her go.

This bonding process repeats itself over and over again, every single day. The process starts with
the parents and continues later on in relation to brothers, sisters, grandfathers, grandmothers,
uncles, aunts, at school and so forth.

This development cycle also involves separation. All bonds eventually lead to a transition
or to an end.

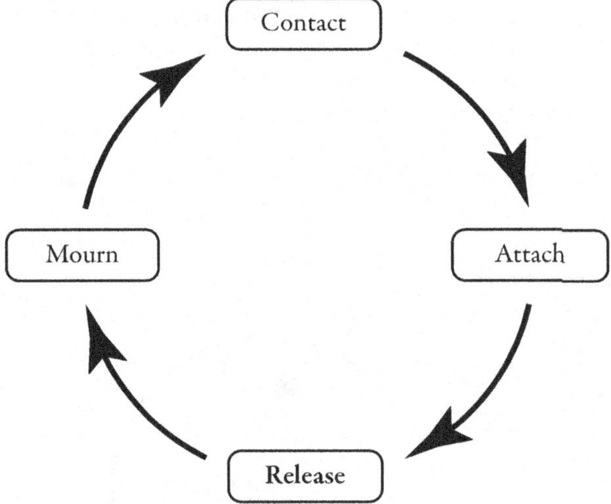

Figure: Attachment - Bonding – Separation – Grief

George Kohlrieser's Cycle of Bonding

If you are able to go through the cycle of bonding in a healthy way as a child, you will be
able to cope with the developmental stages in life.

Assignment

Take a look at a relationship you, at some point in time, have finalised at work or in your private situation, in terms of the cycle of bonding.

> **How did you connect?**
> **How did you get attached to this person? Think of some practical examples.**
> **Did you say goodbye? How?**
> **Did you grieve? How?**
> **Visualise the role of the other person while you think of these four steps.**
> **What do you see?**
> **Were you able to connect with another person later on?**
> **Which of these steps do you easily manage?**
> **Which steps do you find hard?**

The Stages of Development

A healthy bonding offers a secure base for us to grow and develop. Ideally speaking, this development follows a shared set of patterns of growth. Pamela Levin called this the 'cycle of development'. In this continuing cycle throughout our lives, Levin distinguishes several recurrent stages:

1.   The power of Being
2.   The power of Doing
3.   The power of Thinking
4.   The power of Identity
5.   The power of Skills
6.   The power of Integration
7.   The power of Recycling

The basis for development lies in the primary bonding of a child.

These stages of development are illustrated in the figure at the top of page 8.

As we move through life from birth to death, we respond to an internal developmental clock or organisational pattern that prescribes the tasks and skills we need to learn.

In order to get a better understanding of this cycle, I will illustrate the various stages by using examples that occur in early childhood and in later stages in life.

1   The power of Being (0 to 6 months)

I saw my second cousin Ziva for the first time yesterday. She was just one week old. She was sound asleep in her cot. Her tiny fisted hands were raised above her head. Her mother told me that she only slept and ate.

The first stage of our life is all about Being. Being only concerns experiencing the world. At this stage, a baby will need to eat, drink, sleep, be comfortable and be

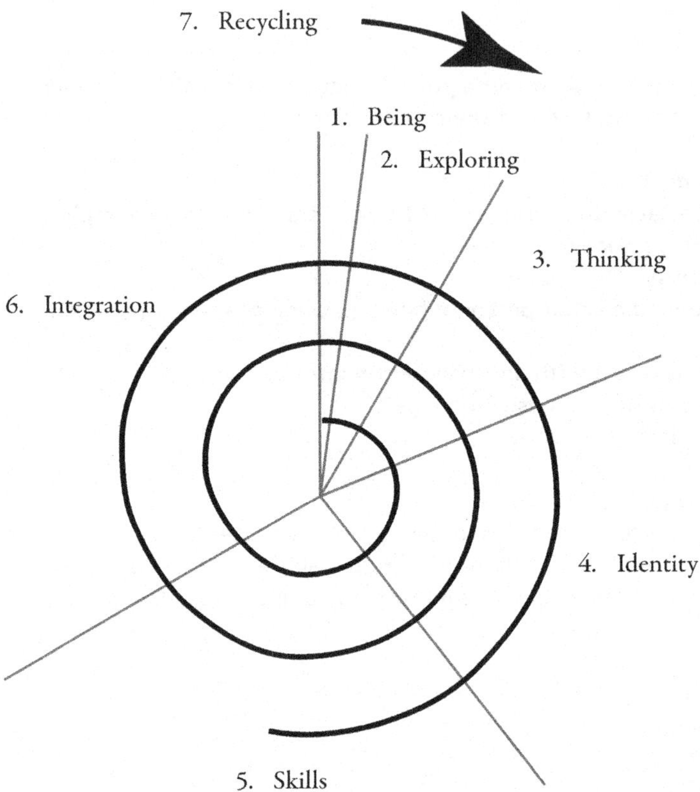

The Stages of Development

held. When a baby is given all these things, it will develop a sense of trust knowing that its surroundings will meet its needs. From there on the child will develop the ability to connect with others and itself.

Frank was exhausted after his first day at work in his new job. He hadn't done anything. 'He had merely been there.' He had shaken hands and had gained many new impressions. It was all very different in this new workplace and he needed to get used to the new situation.

2   The power of Doing (6 to 18 months)

David is exploring the world. Sometimes his parents would like to tie him down. He creeps and crawls across the entire room, grabs things and puts everything he gets hold of into his mouth.

The second stage is about Doing. Children explore their world through their senses: they smell, touch, look, listen and taste. They are seeking sensations that give them pleasure, they experience pain and do new things. They have a short attention span due the huge amount of stimuli they receive.

At the first weeks in his new job, Frank feels like he is on a roller coaster. Every day he is learning to do new things: getting in touch with the bank's clients, his first home visit for a mortgage, his first meeting with colleagues. It's all new, exciting and energising for him to do. At last he feels he is able to bring into practice what he has been trained to do.

3 The Power of Thinking (18 months to 3 years)

The little boy flings himself onto the floor in the middle of the supermarket and starts screaming: 'I want that bag of sweets!' His mother stays calm, kneels by the side of her son and tells him gently that he is allowed to pick out a bag of sweets another time. After a short while, the little boy gets up, wipes his nose and says: "May I choose the next time"?

During this life stage children develop their thinking skills. They start seeing themselves as separate beings from their parents. They will want to reason things out for themselves and make their own decisions. They do that by testing the limits of their parents and resisting parental demands. In this phase we start to develop our own unique character.

Frank has been working at the bank for about three months. He has received sufficient on the job training. Gradually he notices that things aren't always going the way he would like them to go. He believes, for instance, that the customer calls procedure could be improved. He decides to discuss this with his boss. His boss listens and gives him space to experiment.

4 The power of Identity (3 to 6 years)

Eliza sits down next to her father on the couch with a very serious expression on her face. 'What happens when you die?', she asks. In response to his detailed answer she asks: 'Why are the clouds white?'.

In this stage in life children develop their own identity. During the process they ask a lot of questions about how the world works. Based on the way they take things in, they will make decisions as to their place in their family and their place within the bigger picture.

Frank really gets going after successfully creating his own procedure. He often consults his boss asking him about the 'how and why' of rules and regulations within the bank. Sometimes his boss gets tired of this. After he explains, Frank appears to be satisfied. However, just as Frank walks out of the door, he pops his head around the corner wanting to share an idea which he introduces by saying: "But wouldn't it be better if . . . ?"

5 The Power of Skills (6 to 12 years)

That day, Anna's mother let Anna and her friend go the grocery store by themselves. Standing in front of the store, Anna's friend suggests to buy sweets instead of the groceries and then to act as if they have lost the money. No sooner said than done. Once they get home Anna tells her mother that they lost the money. Her mother stays calm and asks them to go and look for the money. Eventually Anna bursts out into tears and tells her mother what had really happened.

The most important task in this stage is to learn skills and to develop a personal value system. In this phase it is important to have conversations with others and (be allowed) to make mistakes and learn from them.

In the meantime Frank has become quite a successful mortgage broker. One day his boss knocks on his door and points out to him that he has given a family reason to believe that they could get a mortgage that should actually be denied. Frank argues that it could be possible by bending the rules a bit. His boss then argues back that his concern is not about bending the rules, but whether or not the family could get into trouble in future.

6 The power of Integration (13 to 18 years)

As if overnight, Steven has turned from a boy into a young man. He is tall and almost as big as his father. Girls are noticing him and he notices the girls. He manages his life the way he wants to. And sometimes he gets close to his father and leans against him when they watch a scary movie together.

In this stage the important task of adolescents is to weave the various parts of their own personality into a coherent whole. Here the young person will recycle through all the previous stages of development again and gradually create their own views on life. This goes hand in hand with rapid physical changes and the development of a sexual identity of our own.

In the meantime Frank has become a financial advisor at the bank. He executes all his work independently, without consulting others. But sometimes he encounters a complex and challenging situation. This often occurs when questions arise of a more personal nature. He then goes over to his boss' office and asks his boss to help him out.

7 The power of Recycling

After five years of working at the bank Frank reaches the level of senior advisor and gets a transfer to another branch of the bank. On his first day at work he goes into his new office, full of confidence. When he arrives home late in the evening he is exhausted. He hadn't done a thing. He feels that 'he had only been there', meeting a lot of new people, shaking hands and gaining many new impressions. In this branch things are totally different and it will take some getting used to.

Assignment

Can you identify the stage of development you are at now with regard to work?
And which stage in your private life?
How can you tell? Talk to others about it. They often have a clearer view.
Could there be stages in which you might get stuck?

During our lives we repeat this cycle every time we enter into a new life task. But also when the change in our lives is smaller, we go through the various stages in much shorter time. As described, each stage has its own development task. If you have accomplished a development task successfully in an earlier stage of life, you will have the ability to deal with this task in a flexible way when it recurs in a later stage in your life (recycling).

In case, for whatever reason, you haven't been able to fulfil this development task in earlier stages, you will encounter the consequence of this later on in life. There are various ways to deal with this. You can either hide your inability from yourself and others by putting on a mask, or you can decide to accomplish the development task now. During your life you will find that there are opportunities to go through each development stage over and over again up to the point that you fully utilise your potential.

Sandra has been together with Carl for fifteen years now. After leaving her parent's house, she moved straight in with him. Suddenly she has enough of shadowing him, the same way she had followed her father when she was young. She wants to make her own decisions and manage her own affairs. Carl has difficulty with that, especially because, from his point of view, she can be 'unreasonable in doing so'. In relationship talks with their counsellor, Carl and Sandra both learn the importance for each partner to stand on his or her own feet and also to give each other the personal space that is required. They also learn the importance of mutual support by acknowledging each other in a positive way.

When you want to develop new behaviours, it is important that you give yourself acknowledgment for this and that people in your environment support, praise and encourage you on your way. This often will give you the boost to do things differently. You can receive and give this acknowledgment in various ways: a compliment, a pat on the back, a greeting card, a gift. You can ask for this acknowledgment and you can give it to yourself. Don't be modest: there is more than enough to go around.

In case you don't receive the acknowledgment, chances are you will fall back into your old habits and patterns and pull out your mask to wear again. You will be confirmed in your belief that there is no alternative. Changing the way you behave will be hard.

Jim decides to stop bullying his biology teacher and starts paying attention in class. His classmates interpret Jim's new behaviour as a sign of weakness and the teacher doesn't even appear to be noticing that he was being quiet and paying attention. When his teacher sends him out of the classroom for something he hasn't done, Jim decides that his new attitude is not making a real difference and he starts joining in with his friends bullying the teacher again.

You start wearing your mask again when you fall back into your old habits and patterns.

Second Act: Masks and Make-up: the camouflage of life

3. Ego-states

It is a wise father that knows his own child.

William Shakespeare, 'The Merchant of Venice', Act 2, Scene 2

In the previous chapter I described Pamela Levin's 'Cycle of development'. Moving through the seven stages of development in a healthy way will evolve into a healthy personality. Although I believe that the whole idea of 'moving through stages in a healthy way' may be interpreted lightly, in all families children take something of a knock. Little cracks and dents form our personality. I will get back to that when explaining about script in Chapter 6.

In this chapter I will talk about ego-states. Ego-states – a core concept of Transactional Analysis - provide a way of *understanding our personality*; how we think, feel and behave. With this model it is possible to investigate many different parts of your own personality. You can use it to look at the various kinds of messages and experiences that have shaped you. You can also investigate how these messages and experiences still influence your behaviour and how this affects your communication with others. The ego-state model is also a powerful tool you can use to change your communication style for the better. In this chapter I will explain what ego-states are and how they develop.

What Are Ego-States?

The basic model of ego-states is used within TA to symbolise the different parts of our personality: a consistent pattern of feeling, thinking and experience directly related to a corresponding consistent pattern of behaviour.

A 'major' definition that needs to be chewed on! You could consider ego-states as ways or modes of being, ways in which we relate to our environment whilst our thinking, our feeling and our actions are logically coherent.

This model of ego-states can be extremely useful when you wish to understand your own behaviour, the behaviour of other(s) and also to find out what is actually happening when you interact.

Since its introduction by Eric Berne, three types of ego-states are distinguished:

the Child
the Adult
the Parent

These three ego-states are always drawn as three circles, one above the other, containing the capital letters P, A and C.

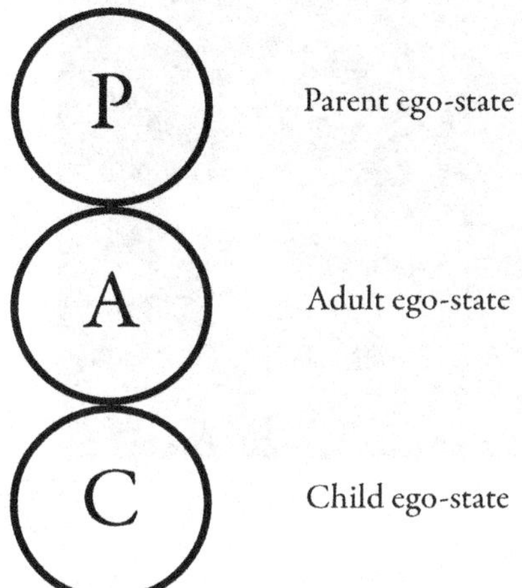

Parent ego-state

Adult ego-state

Child ego-state

The Child

The Child is the ego-state that we have filled with all our own childhood memories and experiences. These memories and experiences are unique for each and every child and form the basis upon which the Child ego-state develops. We learn how to think, feel and behave consistently based on experiences early in life.

Francine (33) has no trouble connecting with her team colleagues. She is cheerful and straightforward. Everybody likes having her around. 'I have infinite trust in people', she tells me. I ask her how come and she describes the warm nest of a happy supportive family she grew up in. 'That's where I learnt to trust people', she decides.

Henry (38) keeps at an almost arrogant distance from all others in the training. When I speak to him in private he tells me how he had always been bullied at school when he was a little boy, and how he gets triggered into a survival mode whenever he is with a group of people.

These two examples illustrate how we carry our childhood experiences along with us in adult life. Often, there are certain experiences we have not been able to deal with as a child and in effect we 'make our own masks' or 'put on make-up' to protect ourselves. Like Henry, who has developed the 'mask of arrogance' in order to keep people at a distance to protect himself from being bullied.

Developmental neurobiology gives us a better understanding of how experience in early life affects our behaviour. Our brain is designed to constantly make and break neural connections and create neural pathways. Neural pathways are like superhighways of nerve cells that transmit messages. You travel over the superhighway many times, and the pathway becomes more and more solid. Like walking down the path that is known to you and that is heavily worn and trodden on from years of use. This explains why we are driven by our experiences.

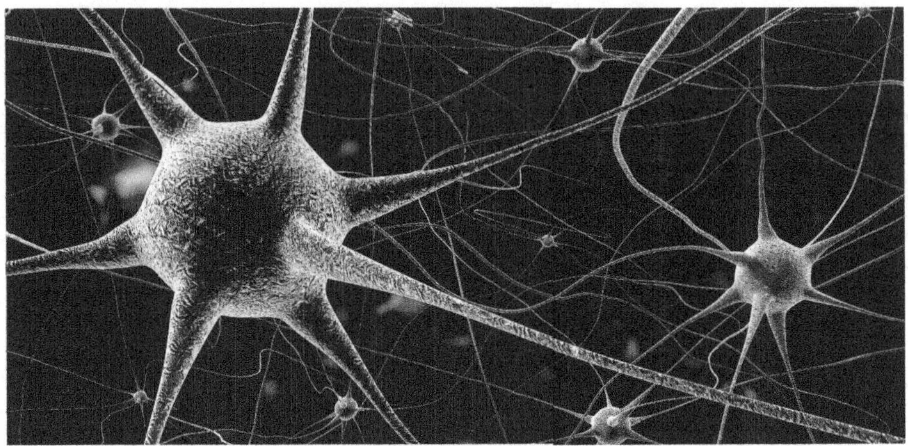

The making and breaking of neural pathways

The Parent

We also tread the worn paths we are so familiar with in another way by following the paths our parents have taken in life. During your childhood, parental figures of importance to you communicated numerous messages to you about how they believe the world works and how you should behave in it. Not only parents play an important role in the upbringing of a child, but also grandfathers and grandmothers, teachers, neighbours, et cetera. All can be seen as influential parent-like figures because of the messages they have transmitted to the child. Each child internalises these messages in its own unique way.

Sandra is a talented theatre producer. In spite of her talent, she has not yet been able to make the production she so much desires. During one of our first conv ersations she tells me about the environment she grew up in: both her parents were talented and smart, but her father remained working in a factory his entire life and her mother ran the household. Together they could barely make ends meet.

This example gives you a better understanding of how we all unconsciously take on certain experiences from our parents, like an inheritance. We store these experiences in what is called the Parent-ego state: thoughts, feelings and behaviour taken from parents and parental figures. This is how experiences and entire life patterns get transferred from generation to generation. We inherit the masks from the past so to speak.

My grandfather passed away at a young age. My grandmother barely had any money and she depended on the church for help. Church charity funding enabled her children to go to school and get an education. One of her sons, my father, was a clever boy who got far in life. After high school, he went to university. Time and again he had to submit his school results to the Church Council who would only continue to fund his education if he was able to get high grades. And he succeeded. As a consequence, during his entire life, my father loathed authorities. I copied this aversion blindly. However, this aversion was based on my father's experience, and not on the experience of my own. Yet every time I was confronted with authorities, I got into trouble. I automatically got into arguments with them. When I grew older, I realised that I was fighting my father's battle.

You can imagine how behavioural patterns get passed on from generation to generation without us even being aware of their origin. The following amusing anecdote may illustrate this:

Whenever Hank was cooking roast meat, he sliced it in half before putting it in the oven. His girlfriend was curious to know why he did this. When she asked Hank he shrugged his shoulders and said that it was the way it was supposed to be done. That was how his mother had taught him to do it. His girlfriend couldn't settle for that answer, so she went to ask Hank's mother the same question. His mother gave her the same answer: 'That's the way it's supposed to be done, that's how my mother taught me to do it.' Still not satisfied she went to ask Hank's grandmother who gave her the clarifying answer: 'In the early days we had to slice the meat in half because we didn't have a pan big enough to roast it in.'

Assignment

Write down two notable behaviours you believe you have taken from your parents.

> **How did your parents learn this kind of behaviour and in which way have they passed it on to you?**
> **How have these (their) experiences influenced your behaviour up till this day and age?**
> **Which situations trigger you into this kind of behaviour?**
> **What kind of behaviour do you then display?**
> **What name would you give this mask?**

The Adult

We also have access to the Adult ego-state in which we are able to check reality from the most objective perspective possible. Whilst the Child and the Parent fill themselves with our own earlier experiences and those of others, the Adult makes choices how to respond in the here-and-now; thoughts, feelings and behaviour are a direct response to what is happening in the here-and-now.

John tells me how he has recently solved a crisis at work. 'Sometimes I can be very indecisive, but in this situation I knew exactly what had to be done. I gave my team instructions and gave my superior the necessary information and acted in a flow. The whole time I felt determined and confident. It felt wonderful not to be hindered by any old heritage.

The Adult anticipates how to respond to the situation that is presented and is not obstructed by experiences form the past. When your Adult ego-state is 'turned on' you are able to assess the situation clearly and to respond effectively in a number of appropriate ways: you can either choose to structure, nurture, cooperate or use your creativity or choose to apply a combination of these behaviours.

Assignment

Describe two recent experiences you are very happy about because you were able to act in an effective and successful way.

> **What were you feeling, thinking and doing?**
> **How come you were able to behave in an effective and successful way?**

In the Adult ego-state we are able to respond in the here-and-now, but that doesn't mean to say that our behaviour is actually derived from the here-and-now. We have learnt most of our behaviour earlier in life. Yet we are able to take off our mask and choose freely how we want to behave and assess whether or not this behaviour suits the situation in front of us.

Patrick, a successful business manager, tells me that he finds it easier to run his business than to manage his son. 'My son is becoming more independent and is going his own way. But whenever I don't know what he's up to, I feel anxious. And then I get angry, almost violent.' During our conversation it becomes clear to Patrick that his reactions are similar to the way his father used to react towards him. Patrick was currently reacting from the Parent-ego state towards his son. He was unconsciously following the imprint of one of his father's deeply ingrained habits. He had to become aware of this pattern before he was able recognise his capacity to apply options and choose autonomously how to react in the here-and-now whilst making use of the Adult ego-state.

Patrick has recently spoken with his son. 'I told him that I wasn't always behaving in a desirable way towards him because of my concern and fear that something bad might happen to him. We talked it over. My son understands and he has promised to keep me posted on his activities and his whereabouts. I told him that this would make it easier for me to let go of him. And do you know what? It works. This week my son even came to me for a bit of advice!'

We can take off the mask.

4. In conversation with Ego-states

The course of true love never did run smooth.

William Shakespeare, 'A Midsummer Night's Dream', Act 1, Scene 1

In the previous chapter, I explained the structure of personality using ego-states. In this chapter I will describe how ego-states work when in contact with other people and how ego-states interact from one person to the other. This may help you become more aware of your own patterns of communication and also help you explore how you could change these patterns to your own and others' benefit. In order to explain I will make use of an extensive version of the ego-state model, the so-called functional model of ego-states. In this model (see below), distinctions are made within the various ego-states.

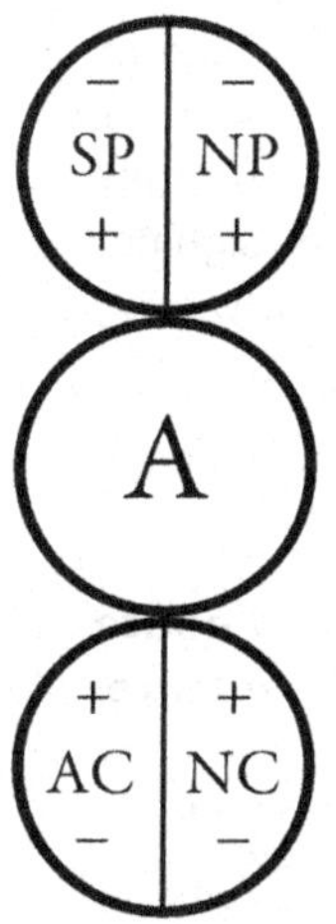

The Parent is divided into:

a.   The Structuring Parent (SP) – in this position you can offer useful structure, guidance and limitations. In the negative mode you can be critical and dominant towards others.

b.   The Nurturing Parent (NP) – in this position you can be caring, supportive and understanding towards others. In the negative mode you can be patronising, suffocating, and over-anxious.

The Child is divided into:

a.   The Adapted Child (AC) – in this position you can cooperate with others. In the negative mode you can be either over-adapted or rebellious.

b. The Natural Child (NC) – in this position you can experience your emotions, be playful and energetic. In the negative mode you can behave in an immature, egocentric, childish or reckless way.

The Parent and Child ego-states both have a positive and a negative side from which we respond out of awareness. We are led by past experiences and examples we have copied and internalised into habits. These habits have been deeply ingrained to the extent that we often act automatically.

Assignment

Take the Structuring and the Nurturing Parent in mind and think of a positive and a negative example from your own life.
Do the same for the Adapted and Natural Child.
How were you behaving? How were others behaving?

Transactions

The last question above is about how you communicate with others and how your behaviour invites others to respond in a certain way and vice versa. In TA this kind of communication between people is called transactions. Transactions are units, or fragments, within a pattern of communication between people. People constantly communicate with each other in many ways: speaking, exchanging glances, sighing, groaning or making gestures. We also exchange different kinds of messages by varying in the tone, pitch, rhythm, timbre and volume of our voice.

Assignment

Read the sentence 'I'm reading this book' out loud in various ways and notice how the meaning changes when different words are stressed in the sentence. Find out how it sounds when you say it:

questioningly
critically
enthusiastically

Look in the mirror:

What changes can you see in your facial expressions?
What changes are there in your voice?
Can you feel a difference in muscle strain?

Transmitter and Receiver

There are two roles to be played in a transaction: that of the transmitter and that of the receiver.

The receiver of the message is always the one who gives meaning to the message. The receiver interprets the meaning of the message partly by what you say. But the biggest part of meaning is conveyed by implicit messages, whether intentional or not, which are expressed through non-verbal behaviours. The receiver will then respond on the basis of their interpretation of the meaning and in turn will become the transmitter.

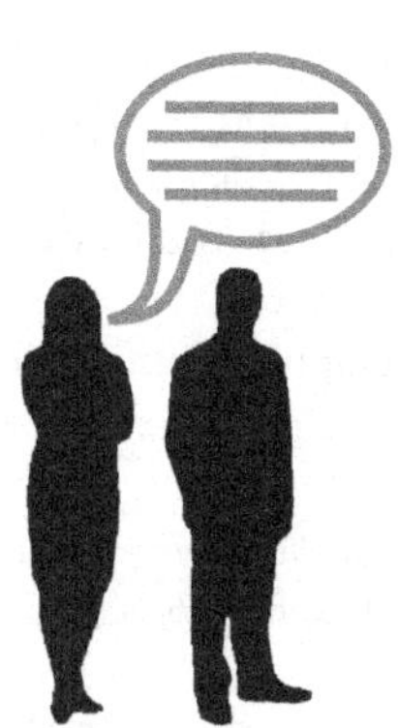

He: Could you clear the table before our visitors arrive?
She: Why do you always have to growl at me?

In this example she gives a negative connotation to his question. Her interpretation of the meaning can be based on:

the content of the question
the tone of voice and volume
his look
his gestures
her own past experience (for example her mother who always asked her to do things with a critical tone of voice)

It is the tone that makes the music
The fact of the matter is that it is not so much **what** you say that is of importance, but **how** you say it. And that is why communication is extremely complex. Or you could also say it's extremely fascinating because so many elements are involved.

Can you recall a situation in which you were misunderstood by another person?

What was your message?
How was it received?
How did you convey your message?

Transaction Patterns
For a better understanding of communication between people, Transactional Analysis (the analysis of transactions) distinguishes various kinds of transactions:

The complementary transaction – in this transaction people respond to each other in an anticipated pattern. B invites A to respond in a certain way and A responds accordingly.

The crossed transaction – in this transaction people respond differently than what is expected. This unexpected response can be seen as an invitation to the transmitter to change the transaction pattern.

The transaction with an ulterior motive – in this transaction pattern people say something that isn't congruent with what they are communicating with their tone of voice and gestures. They are then conveying two different messages.

These transaction patterns can help you investigate how you communicate to others and vice versa. More importantly, once you understand you will be able to influence communication patterns between yourself and others.

To get a picture of your transactions, you can make use of the functional model of ego-states. In the following examples I will show you how the various transaction patterns work, taking into consideration that the sound of the voices, the volume, et cetera, are lacking. You'll just have to imagine how things are said.

Complementary Transaction
A complementary transaction may resemble the following example:

Mother: Robert, finish your plate. (Structuring Parent (SP) inviting Robert to respond from Adapted Child (AC)); this is a SP-AC transaction. Robert: Yes mum. (AC-SP).

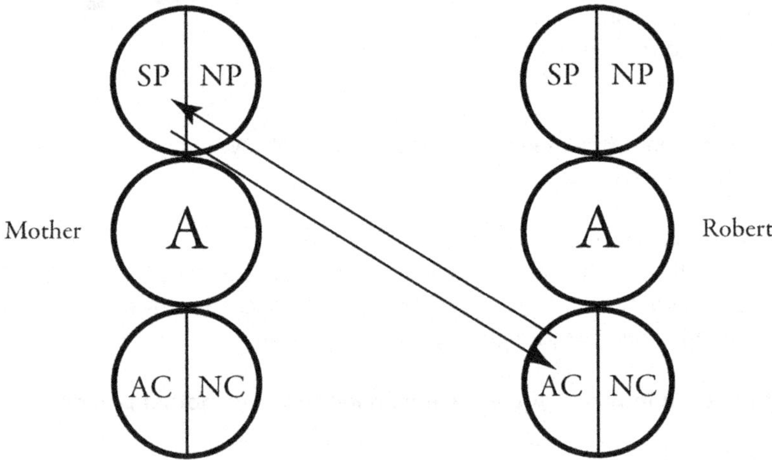

The figure above shows how a complementary transaction can take place. The mother addresses Robert's Adapted Child and he responds by obeying. Robert and his mother have complementary behaviour towards each other. Both mother and son 'agree' as to 'who should be in which ego-state'. This communication pattern can continue indefinitely, as long as the transaction remains complementary.

Another example:

John: Are you just as excited as I am about going to the concert tonight? (NC – NC)
Ellen: Absolutely, I can't wait. (NC – NC).

This example illustrates how John and Ellen share how much they are looking forward to the concert that evening. They too are complementary in the way they communicate with each other.

These examples might be confusing you. You don't need to force yourself to comprehend it all immediately. That will probably only lead to frustration. What is of importance now is that you are becoming aware of the fact that you are able to respond in many different ways.

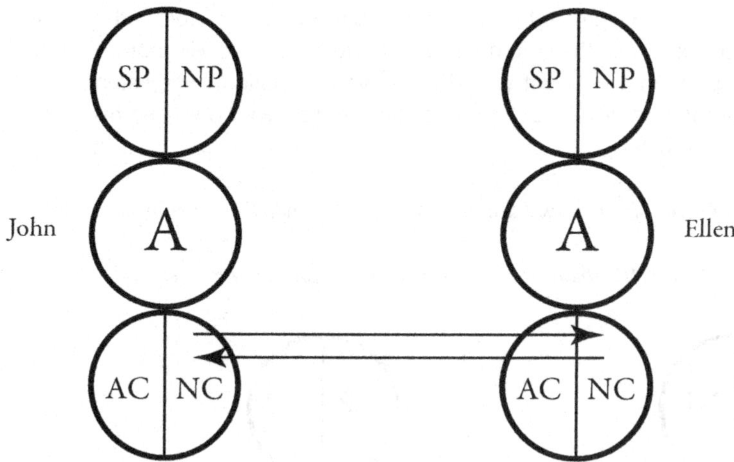

Assignment

Think of examples of complementary transactions that you recognise in your own situation in terms of:

SP – SP
NP – NP
NP – NC

Crossed Transaction

The following example is slightly more complex:

Mother: Robert, finish your plate. (SP – AC)
Robert: Mum, I'm 18 years old. I think I am able to decide for myself whether or not to finish my plate. (A – A).

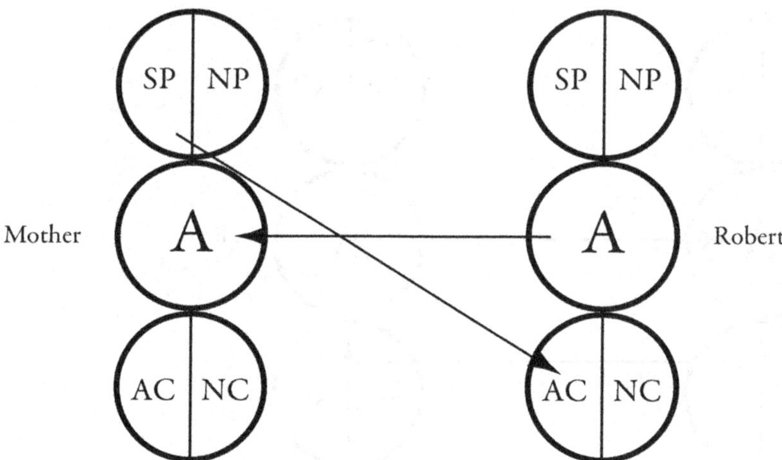

Robert's transaction is called a crossed transaction; Robert's response crosses that of his mother's and as a consequence the communication pattern changes. His mother is now being invited to respond in a different way. She has various options. For instance, she can say: 'You're right Robert. It's about time I let you stand on your own two feet.' This transaction is illustrated below:

Robert: Mum, I'm 18 years old. I think I am able to decide for myself whether or not to finish my plate. (A – A).
Mother: You're right Robert. It's about time I let you stand on your own two feet. (A - A)

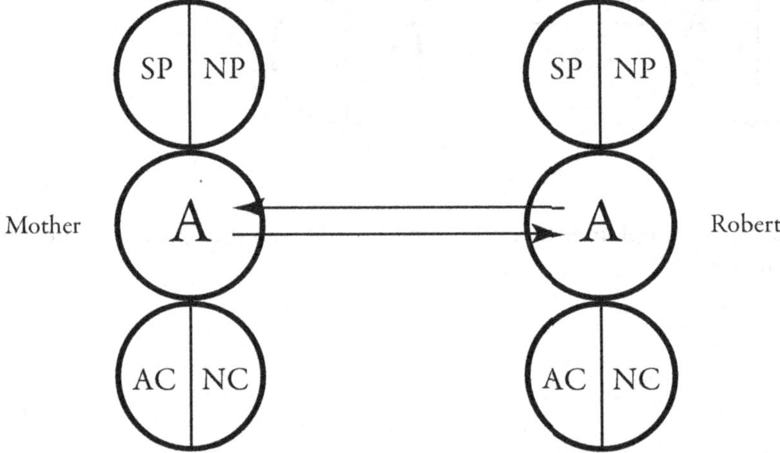

In this case the mother decides to answer with a complementary transaction. Let's take a look at how this works using John and Ellen's example.

John: Are you just as excited as I am about going to the concert tonight? (NC – NC)
Ellen: I'll start thinking about that after I've done my work. (A – A)

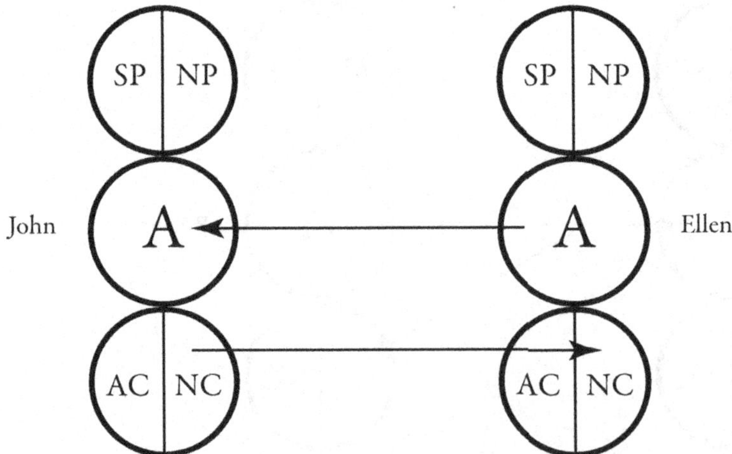

John also has various response options. He could say: 'You're right, I have some chores to do myself.' This transaction looks like this:

Ellen: I'll start thinking about that after I've done my work. (A – A)
John: 'You're right, I have some chores to do myself.'

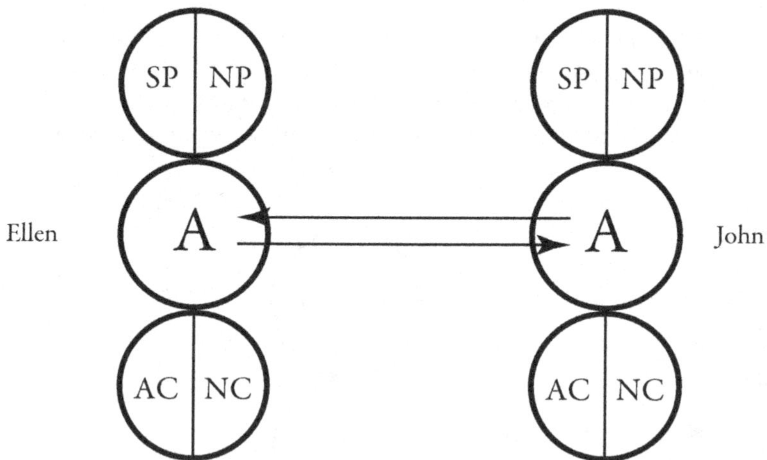

John also chooses to respond with a complementary transaction.

Assignment

Imagine John choosing to respond with a crossed transaction.

> **What are his options?**
> **Can you think of sentences to match the various options?**
> **And how could Ellen then respond?**
> **What kind of transaction would that be?**

Again, at this stage it is more important for you to play with the models and enjoy discovering than it is to get results. I'm inviting you to explore the incredible amount of options you have.

Ulterior Transactions

Robert's mother could also have answered in another and much more complex way by saying: *'Robert, you can't do without me, can you?' (A – A at social level, but something else at the psychological level.*

This example reveals the various levels on which communication can take place. One of the levels is called the social level, which is based on what is actually being said. The other level is called the psychological level, which is based on all other aspects of communication mentioned earlier, such as tone of voice, volume and glance. In the previous examples, these levels of communication were congruent. The spoken message at social level matched what was being communicated at psychological level.

However, in this example, Robert's mother conveys the message on two different levels: at social level the message is overt with the use of words. On psychological level, she is conveying a totally different message in a muffled way.

What if the mother had communicated the message with a slight tremor in her voice and sad eyes? This is how I imagined her saying it when I thought of this example (AC – NP). The message would have been conveyed in a completely different way if the mother had said it with a surprised look on her face and a slightly arrogant tone in her voice (SP – AC).

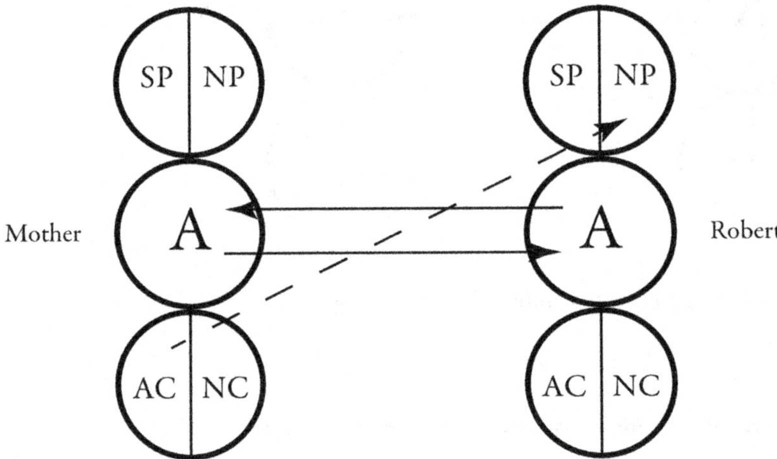

The message that is transmitted at the psychological level will determine the result of the transaction.

The mother might be speculating Robert's response to be: 'No, of course not mum.' And then the communication pattern will go back to how it was before.

Let's take a look at John and Ellen and see what can happen when a similar sequence of transactions occurs between them. Suppose Ellen says to John: 'Good job getting your priorities straight now.'

This is how the transaction could continue:

John: you're right, I have some chores to do myself. (A – A)
Ellen: Good job getting your priorities straight (A – A at social level, but SP – AC at psychological level).

Ellen's response could then trigger John at the psychological level: 'Trust you to get all critical again!'

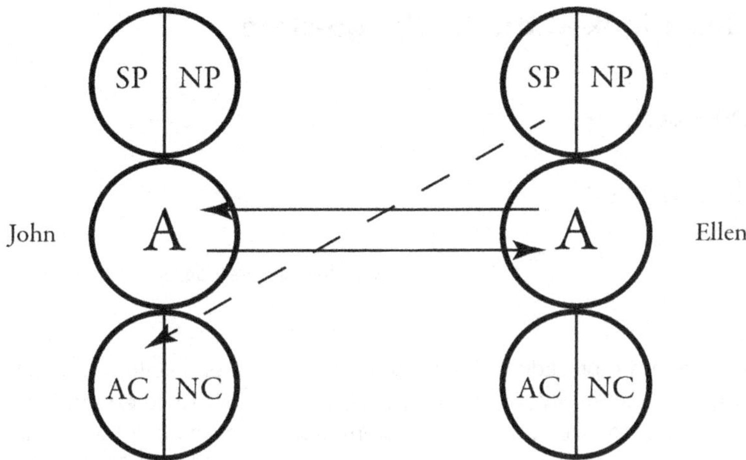

Assignment

> If you give words to the hidden message Robert's mother is transmitting,
> which words would you choose?
> And which words would you choose to describe Ellen's message to John?
> What kind of feelings do these sentences evoke?
> How would you respond?

Three Rules of Communication

Looking back at the previous examples, three important rules of communication can
be derived:

> As long as transactions remain complementary, communication can continue
> indefinitely.
> When a transaction is crossed, a break in communication results and one or both
> individuals will need to shift ego-states in order for communication to be re-established.
> The behavioural outcome of an ulterior transaction is determined at the
> psychological and not at the social level.

Assignment

Think of a recent conversation that left you amazed.

> **From which ego-state were you communicating?**
> **And the person you were having the conversation with?**
> **Can you recall if you switched to another ego-state during the conversation?**
> **If so, what made that happen?**

*It is amazing how many transactions you have at
your disposal.*

5. Taking a closer look at the Adult ego-state

Take each man's censure,

but reserve thy judgment.

William Shakespeare, 'Hamlet', Act 1, Scene 3

You may recall reading in the preceding chapter that, of all three ego-states, only the Adult responds to the here-and-now. The Adult is not based on early Child experiences or experiences that have been taken on from the Parent. It must be said that the Parent and Child ego-states are of enormous importance to us during our childhood. They guide us through life when growing up. As youngsters, we do not yet have sufficient knowledge, awareness, experience and tools enabling us to make considered choices. So we learn behaviour shown to us by our parents and our own experience. The masks and cosmetics initially help us find our way through life's complexity and challenges.

In a later stage, when our brain and personality have matured, our ability increases to integrate old experiences and to give them new meaning. Our Adult ego-state is able to play a bigger role, whilst increasingly leaving the automatic Child and Parent reflexes behind us.

Eva has got to the age of 18. Not so long ago she abided by the regime of her parents. Nowadays she thinks things over, mainly by herself, and makes her own choices in daily life.

An extremely important theme of this book is about developing the Adult ego-state. Leading your life from this ego-state enables you to experience things with awareness and to consciously choose your behaviour instead of being led by automatic reflexes.

Example:
When Sandra gets home she notices that Peter hasn't bothered to tidy up the house. The children's toys and clothes are lying around all over the place. She can hear Peter and the little ones laughing upstairs. She feels irritated and angrily makes her way to the stairs planning to go up and teach him a lesson (SP). She foresees that she will be the one doing all the tidying up.

Then she remembers the conversation she and Peter recently had with their social worker and she decides to count to ten. She sits down calmly and imagines what Peter's intentions could be and she also investigates her own needs. When Peter comes down she asks how his day has been. With great enthusiasm Peter tells her about all the fun he and the kids have been having and that they were rather excited. He also apologises for the fact that he hasn't cleared up. Sandra tells him she understands and offers to give him a hand straight after she has told him about her day.

Sandra is very particular about tidiness in the house. This is what her mother had taught her because for her mother, this was the most important thing in the world. 'As long as the house is clean and tidy.' Although Sandra knows that this is totally over the top, she finds it almost impossible to let go of the image of a clean and tidy house. Due to this deeply ingrained belief, Sandra almost automatically gets furious at the sight of a messy house. And this is causing a lot of tension in her relationship with Peter. They are now learning to respond in a different way instead of letting their responses be determined by their old behavioural patterns. In order to do this, they need to 'switch on' their Adult ego-state so that they can consciously make a choice how to behave.

Parent- and child ego-state guide

us through life during childhood.

The Adult ego-state viewed through a magnifying glass looks approximately like this:

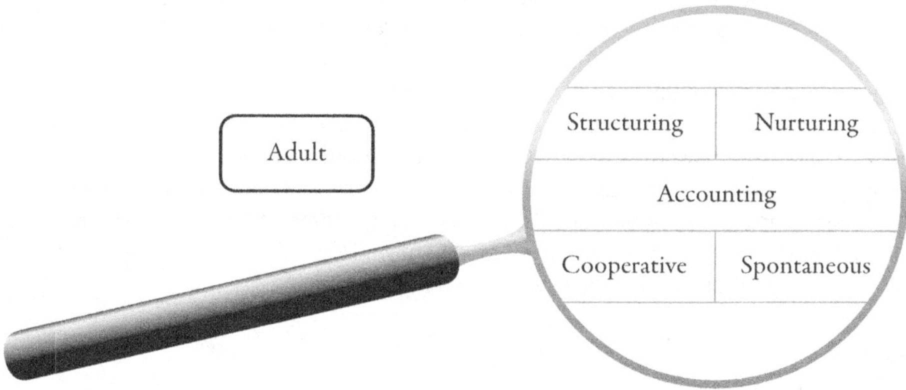

The Adult ego-state viewed through a magnifying glass

When acting from the Adult ego-state you are prepared **to be accountable** for your own behaviour and look at what is needed. Contrary to the automatic reaction from either Parent or Child, you evaluate and investigate your options and consider what to do. Balancing options, you then decide what to do and how to do it, knowing that you have access to a large behavioural repertoire.

You can choose to **structure**, empowering others by guiding and inspiring them and enabling their success.

You can choose to **nurture**, responding to the need of others, offering empathy and encouragement.

You can choose to be **cooperative**, collaborating equally with others, being friendly, paying attention to what is of importance to you and being prepared to adjust to others.

You can choose to follow your own **spontaneity**, giving yourself ample space to be creative, playful and zestful.

Assignment

Can you recall the two situations you described previously when you were very satisfied with your own effective behaviour (Chapter 3, last exercise)? Which of the above-mentioned behaviours were you applying?

In the former example, Sandra decides first of all to connect with Peter by sharing his pleasure about the children and then sharing her day with him, after which she was able to tidy things up together with Peter without an effort. At that point she was no longer being hindered by her mother's messages from the past. She uses her power to cooperate (in connection), to nurture (by listening and paying attention to Peter's story) and give space to her own spontaneity (by sharing Peter's pleasure about the children).

Responding by way of Adult ego-state, she invites Peter to do the same. Not so long ago he used to walk away and sulk when Sandra had a go at him. Now he apologises for not tidying up the house and then takes responsibility by doing it later.

An Intermezzo About Learning

I would like to focus very briefly on the subject of 'learning'. Very often I hear people object by saying that having to think with awareness about your behaviour the whole time will lead to artificial behaviour. Maybe you had the same thought whilst you were reading the example about Sandra and Peter. If so, I quite understand, because in general we are not used to being aware of the way we behave. However, it is still necessary to go through this phase if you want to learn new things.

Assignment

**Can you remember how you cycled when you were just learning to ride a bike?
And how you were driving when you were just learning to drive a car?
Can you describe the difference between then and now?**

When I'm learning new things, I always find it helpful to keep the learning curve in mind.

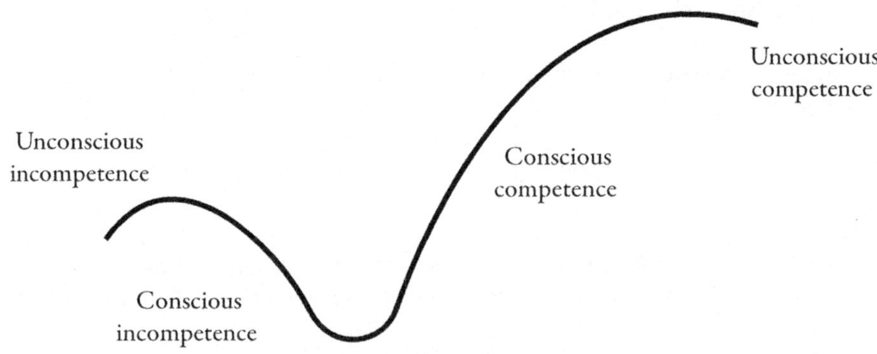

There are various claims about the source of this model and it seems likely that it goes back to an ancient oriental proverb that has been given some catchy labels.

Let me walk you through the various stages of the learning process:

Unconscious incompetence – you do not understand or know how to do something, but it doesn't bother you. Maybe you don't even recognise the deficit. *When I was 30, I couldn't drive a car. I always travelled by train. It didn't bother me one bit that I wasn't able to drive. And I was totally unaware of what driving a car entailed.*

Conscious incompetence – you do not understand or know how to do something and this bothers you. You feel awkward about it. *At the age of 31, I started to take driving lessons. My work was increasingly taking me to places afar and I needed a car. The first lessons were a nightmare. All of a sudden I had to take the wheel, change gears, look in the mirrors and pay attention to the traffic in front of me and behind me. I felt extremely clumsy.*

Conscious competence – you have learned something new, however doing it requires concentration and there is a heavy conscious involvement in executing the new skill. *I was 32 when I passed my driving test and from there on I was allowed to drive independently. This required my full attention.*

Unconscious competence – you have had so much practice with a skill that it has become 'second nature' and you can perform it easily. You don't even have to think about it whilst you're doing it. *I've been driving a car for 17 years now, travelling 15,500 miles per year. I hardly have to think about what I am doing when driving and feel relaxed enjoying listening to music. (although I do of course still pay a lot of attention to what might be happening around the car – it is just that I no longer have to think about changing gears and so on).*

The learning curve reflects the movement in the way you learn to do things. At first you feel incapable, as if you're on a downhill slide. Then you move upwards feeling that you're learning but you are aware that you have to be conscious of each step you take. Eventually you look back in amazement, hardly able to imagine that at one time you felt so incompetent.

Gerald became a manager at a young age. He was experiencing quite some resistance from his employees and he came to me asking how he could learn to deal with it. In the conversations we had, Gerald found out that his competitive drive had helped him to achieve a leadership position, but that this drive was no longer serving him as a leader. If he were to overcome his employees' resistance, he had to learn that 'being the best' wouldn't contribute to solving the problem. More importantly, in this stage, was the necessity for him to let his employees feel that he trusted them. One of the assignments I gave him was to set himself the task of giving his employees at least three compliments every day. At first he moaned and groaned about having to do this exercise. 'It feels so artificial.' After I had explained to him that this is what life is about, he agreed to take serious action. I encouraged him to just take notice of the effect his compliments were having on his employees. He started doing it and after a while he told me: 'It really makes them happy.'

Gerald learned especially by paying attention to how he connected with his employees.

A significant question to ask yourself is: 'Am I connected?' Followed by the question: 'What can I do to connect (even) more deeply?' These questions are keys to behavioural change.

Journey of Life
Basically, the life journey of all people is about gradually responding less and less from Parent and Child, doing away with their masks by increasingly using the Adult. Think of the learning curve as a landscape with peaks and valleys, ups and downs. Along the way you integrate all the valuable life experiences, eventually having them all at your disposal in order to choose the behaviour that suits you. You gradually let go of the Parent and Child ego-state. Both have served you well during the first part of your life journey, but are now obstructing you from moving further on. Many of the old messages and behavioural patterns are no longer offering adequate answers to the questions you are currently confronted with.

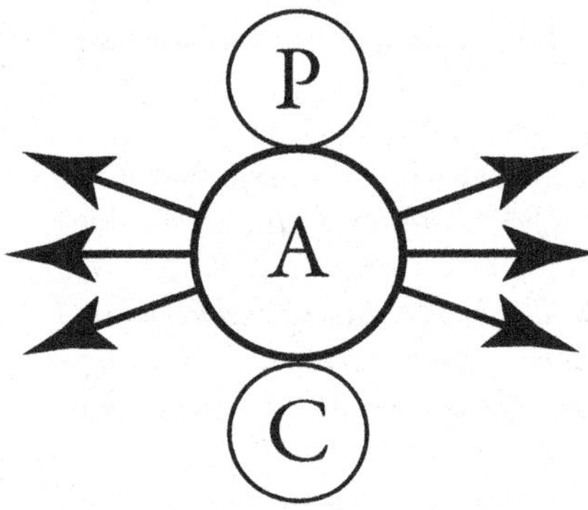

The Adult ego-state expands and the Child and Parent ego-states shrink.

Third Act:
Life Script

6. Script

God hath given you one face

and you make yourselves another.

William Shakespeare, 'Hamlet', Act 3, Scene 1

Introduction

In the previous chapter I discussed the development of ego-states and the way we communicate. Our personal history and how we have experienced things form an important basis for the manner in which we communicate. In order to achieve behavioural change, it is helpful to look back at how your own past history influences your current behaviour. I will elaborate on this in this chapter.

Archaeology is not an end in itself. This 'archaeological' research is only meaningful insofar as it helps you understand the life you are accustomed to and how you can choose to make desirable changes in the (foreseeable) future. Consider this as you complete the questions and exercises in this chapter. Again, you will find that the content is easier to digest when you discuss it with others.

The Script Circle

It follows that the 'content' of ego-states vary per person. Your experiences are not the same as mine and your parents' experiences can't be compared with those of my parents. Basically we can only reflect on the process of how our behaviour is developed. In TA terms this is called development of script; like the progression in a play or film script through beginning and middle to (happy or unhappy) end.

The development of our script consists of a number of recurrent steps:

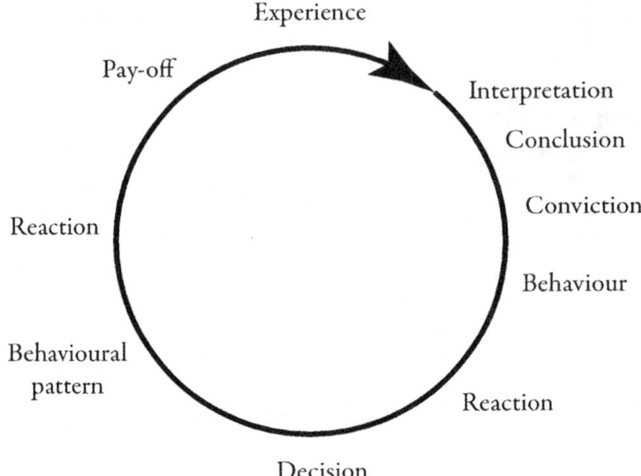

Experience – you have had a significant experience.
Your father is seriously ill and your mother is totally upset and confused.

Interpretation – You give your own meaning to what is happening.
When it comes to the crunch, parents aren't able to take care of themselves.

Conclusion – you come to a conclusion about yourself in this situation.
I have to take care of my parents.

Conviction – your interpretation and conclusion evolve into a conviction.
Because parents are not able to look after themselves, I will have to take care of them.

Behaviour – you start behaving accordingly to your conviction.
Without complaining, you run around cleaning your room, doing the washing up, mowing the lawn and so forth.

Reaction – People around you start responding to your behaviour.
You overhear your mother talking to her neighbour: 'He is doing so well. He is a great support in these difficult times.' And you feel so proud.

Decision – Based on how your environment responds to your behaviour, you take a decision about who and what you are.
In future, I'll take care of everyone who is in need of it.

Behavioural pattern – you act out your decision in all your behaviours.
One of your neighbours falls ill and you start doing her daily groceries. In the meantime you're walking your other neighbour's dog, doing all kinds of chores as well as putting out the rubbish for the entire neighbourhood.

Reaction – your environment responds to your behaviour.

The entire neighbourhood praises you. 'Such a nice boy', 'So grown up and wise for his age' and everyone gives you a friendly nod whenever they see you. Or they give you sweets and some pocket money.

Pay-off – It could be that at some stage in life, you pay the price for all these positive confirmations.
All the kids in the neighbourhood avoid you. They think you're a goody two shoes and they start bullying you.

Interpretation – you start to re-shape your already existing worldview according to this new **Experience**.
Children are cruel. So you're better off being with grown-ups and looking after them, et cetera.

In this process the mask of the 'nurturing, friendly man' takes on a firmer hold. You start arranging your life around this image and as a consequence you camouflage all your anxieties, sadness and anger (towards your parents, your peers) that you are hiding behind the mask.

Assignment

Can you draw your script circle based on an experience you've had or an important decision you've made as to who you want to be in life?

> **Can you describe the experience?**
> **How did you interpret this experience?**
> **What conclusion did you draw about yourself and others?**
> **How did this conclusion influence your behaviour?**
> **How did your environment react?**
> **Which decision did you then make about yourself and others?**
> **In which way did this decision influence your behaviour?**
> **How does your environment respond to your behaviour?**
> **What are the advantages?**
> **What are the disadvantages?**

Rounding up the story

At a young age children tend to look through a magic window at themselves and the world around them when making important decisions about who they are and how they should behave. They interpret all happenings as if they themselves were at the centre of the universe (and many a grown-up does the same). The entirely logical associations children make in their own world are often extremely difficult for grown-ups to comprehend.

He was just able to walk and his mother fastened him with a toddler's belt so that he couldn't run away. He was the only child who was fastened to a belt and for a long time he thought that his mother tied him down because he was such a difficult child. When he was older he talked to his mother about his experience and she explained that at the time she had four youngsters to take care of and that she was afraid that something might happen to him if ever she were to lose him out of sight. He remembers how shocked his mother was after she had learned how he had experienced being tied up.

In addition, children of all ages have the need to make a coherent life story. We interpret events in such a way that they fit into and even reinforce our view of the world. The next example illustrates this.

Twin sisters Jane and Ruth were interviewed on the radio about their experience in the bomb shelter during the bombardment of London. Both girls had the same experience: when the bombs fell, their parents held each other tight. Jane said: 'Seeing my parents hold each other like that made me believe that in times of difficulty, there will always be someone to hold on to.' Ruth responded: 'When I saw my parents holding each other I knew that when it comes down to it, you're on your own.'

Although the bombing was traumatic for both children, they both gave a different meaning to the bomb shelter experience. The way they interpreted the situation could have had far-reaching consequences with regard to the way they were to give meaning to experiences later on in life. Imagine their stories were to continue like this:

Both sisters are in their 70's, both are married and have children. Both become seriously ill. Jane gathers her lov ed-ones around her, tells them about the situation and asks for their support. Every day she receives visitors, flowers and cards. This does her the world of good. She gets confirmed in her old belief that when the going gets rough, there will always be someone there to support you. That's how it has always been in Jane's life.

Ruth hides her illness from others as long as possible up to the point that she can no longer keep it a secret from her husband and children. After telling them about it, she continues to say that she will have no further talk about the matter. She seldom sees her children who only come to visit her out of a sense of duty. She barely speaks with her husband any more. She feels lonely. She gets confirmed in her old belief that when it comes down to it, you're on your own. That's how it has always been in Ruth's life.

Assignment

Go back to your own script circle:

>**In which other way(s) could you have interpreted your experience?**
>**What other kinds of decisions could you have made about yourself and the world around you?**
>**How could the various options have affected your behavioural pattern?**
>**Are you now able to look at the experience from a different perspective?**

Loyalty

Life stories are of all kinds: loveless or loving, boring or full of pleasure, dull or rich in spirit. What all stories have in common is the loyalty towards the parents. This loyalty is about being loyal to your family of origin, your parents and distant family. All know their place. The parents are the parents and the children are the children. This is the way they are connected with each other.

Now and again Karin goes to visit her parents on her own. Her parents love it when Karin is around. Karin enjoys not having to be a mother to her own children for a while and loves the feeling of being her parent's child. In the evening, she sits next to her mother on the couch and rests her head upon her mother's shoulder.

A child's loyalty can go very far to the extent that the child takes on the role of the parent.

Angela's father left home when she was a one-year old. As a child she always felt guilty about him leaving. She thought it was her fault. If she hadn't had been there, her father would have stayed. Now she is older, a middle-aged woman, she goes to visit him once in a while. She is the one who takes the initiative because she feels it is her responsibility to do so.

In order to understand the loyalty of children it is necessary to identify with the child's world. The only world known to the child is the world he grows up in. This is the world the child is accustomed to. In this world he is dependent on his parents and he considers them to be 'good' parents. It would be an immediate threat to his daily life if the child were to think otherwise, in terms of his parents not being 'good'. The blame, if things go wrong, ultimately comes to reside in the child.

Hank's mother started to get migraines immediately after her husband left her. She lay in bed all day with the curtains closed. Hank had taken on the responsibility for his younger brother and sister. One day his little brother fell and broke his arm and Hank felt very guilty. He hadn't looked after his brother properly and now he had disappointed his mother. He was 8 years old at the time.

A small 8-year old boy can't take care of his younger brother and sister. Most adults would agree on that. By not taking her responsibility, Hank's mother was putting a heavy burden on her son. But if you were to put yourself in Hank's shoes, what could be worse: the thought that your mother is not able to cope with life and that she is a bad mother, or the thought that your mother is a good and reliable mother and that you always do the utmost to help and please her.

These loyalty patterns not only repeat themselves towards our own parents, but also in our choices when we find ourselves in similar situations.

Hank is now 35 years old. He still takes care of his mother. He always feels he is failing to meet her needs. He calls on me to be coached. He feels pressured by the way things are going at work, especially the strenuous relationship he has with the business owner. Very often she is ill and she is not able to cope with all the work. Hank does the best he can, but is not able to keep things going. Customers are leaving and sales are dropping. He feels guilty. Especially towards his superior, not being able to do her job.

Assignment

What part does loyalty play in your life towards:

> **your family of origin?**
> **your current family situation?**
> **your work?**

Can you think of an example where loyalty is getting in the way?

Can you think of an example where it is giving you pleasure?

The Influence of The Environment

People are not alone in the world. They are part of groups and social classes. These groups have a big influence in the way we develop our script. They are breeding grounds upon which our script decisions later on in life grow.

Your present behaviour is influenced by your own past.

Assignment

Can you imagine how the following aspects have influenced your script?

> **were you born into an upper class family or a working class family?**
> **did you live in a small or a big house?**
> **did you live in a village or in the city?**
> **was there a lot of noise or was it quiet?**
> **what kind of smells were you familiar with?**
> **were you living in the UK or abroad?**
> **were you a church-going family or not?**
> **are you a boy or a girl?**

Script: Positive or Negative

For years now the question about whether or not a script is positive or negative has caused an on-going discussion within the (international) TA community. Those who see script as something negative argue that script limits you, no matter what. In their point of view, you discount options when in script.

Assignment

Take another look at your script circle: which opportunities have you discounted?

By viewing script in this way, mainly negative and limiting decisions are emphasised. To my way of thinking, I prefer to join Fanita English's positive ideas on script. She argues that script gives you the possibility to blossom. Whatever decisions you have made in life and whatever experiences you have had, they always give you the opportunity to grow and develop.

Take another look at your script circle: which opportunities have your script decisions given you?

7. Components of Script

Though this be madness, yet there is method in it.

William Shakespeare, 'Hamlet', Act 2, Scene 2

In the previous chapter I described how, in general, life scripts are created. In this chapter we will take a closer look at the underlying mechanisms that lead us to make script decisions. This chapter may give you a deeper insight into your own script and how it came to be.

During our upbringing and education we receive numerous messages about how to behave or how not to behave. These messages work like road signs showing us the way: 'You can turn into this road', 'Don't go into that one', 'Prohibited to turn left', 'Only permitted for cars', 'Dead end street'. During early days of childhood we see these signs so often and as a consequence we file them away internally, like on a hard drive of a computer. Eventually, even without hearing the messages, we know what is allowed and what isn't. By putting up the road signs, our parents are helping us develop. They take on certain parts of daily life, as it were, until we are able to take them on ourselves. In the course of this process they teach us who we are.

As a child, Jacob had learned that 'when parents speak, the children must be silent'. From this he concluded that parents are more important than the child.

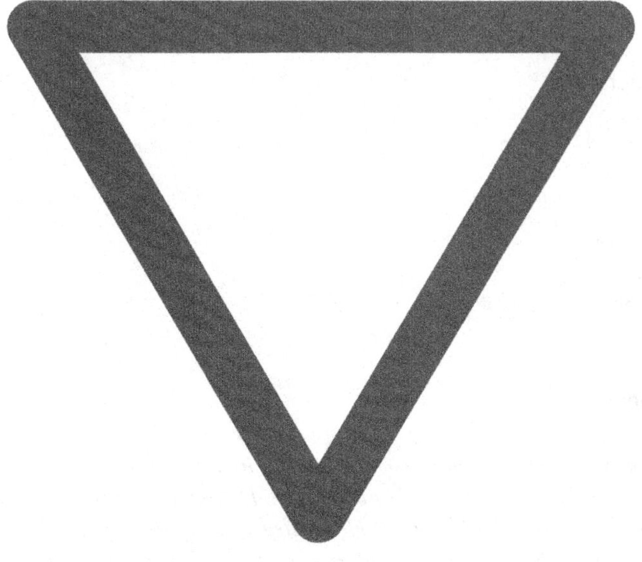

Parents always have right of way

Can you make road signs to illustrate your own upbringing?

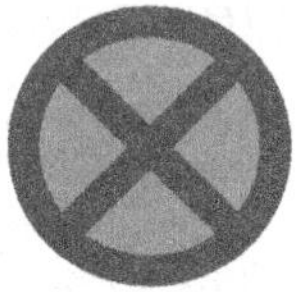

What captions would you give them?

The contents of the messages we receive vary. I will describe the various components in the following order:

> permissions
> injunctions
> driver messages
> program

I will mention a number of messages explicitly. However, it is important to understand that these messages are seldom given in this way to the letter.

Permissions

Children grow when permissions are given. Permissions are positive, comfirmitory messages.

Transactional Analyses distinguishes twelve important themes:

1. You are allowed to exist
2. You are allowed to be yourself
3. You are allowed to grow up
4. You are allowed to be a child
5. You are allowed to succeed
6. You are allowed to do
7. You are allowed to be important
8. You are allowed to belong
9. You are allowed to be close
10. You are allowed to feel
11. You are allowed to think
12. You are allowed to be healthy

The other day I was taking a walk in the woods. A young boy was walking in front of me, together with his grandmother I presumed. Suddenly the boy fell flat on his face. He immediately got on his feet, sniffled a bit and wiped the dirt off his clothes. He 'pulled himself together'. His grandmother kneeled in front of him, took him by his shoulders and said in a gentle voice: It's alright if you want to cry'. The little boy then put his head against her shoulder and started to cry out loud. 15 minutes later I saw him again, running and laughing ahead of his grandmother.

The grandmother gave the boy the permissive message that he was allowed to cry (you are allowed to feel). She holds him close (you are allowed to be close).

Often these permissions are given out of awareness. They are embedded in the parent-child relationship. Often it is only at a later stage that the patterns can be recognised.

Christine is a very popular teacher at College. She pays a lot of attention to her students and encourages them to use their potential to the fullest. During one of our conv ersations I ask her where she had learnt to do that. She smiles and tells me about her mother who always encouraged her to bring out the best in herself and how proud her mother was when she succeeded. She could still hear her mother say: "You're a star!", and how that had made her feel radiant with joy.

Assignment

> **Which permissions can you recall from your own childhood?**
> **What words would you give to them?**
> **Who specifically gave you these permissions?**
> **How do you still benefit from this?**

Injunctions

Injunctions are disallowances. They are the exact opposite of permissions. The following twelve themes can be distinguished:

1. Don't be (Don't exist)
2. Don't be you
3. Don't grow up
4. Don't be a child
5. Don't do anything
6. Don't be important / Don't have needs
7. Don't belong
8. Don't be close
9. Don't feel
10. Don't think
11. Don't be well / Don't be sane
12. Don't make it

You might understandably think this to be quite a harsh list of messages and probably not easy for you to feel within yourself. They need some more explanation.

Injunctions are often about themes that parents haven't (yet) dealt with themselves. Injunctions are parental messages given to them as a child that they in turn have either passed on or transformed into another kind of injunction. Injunctions are passed on from generation to generation, like 'passing on a hot potato' as they say in Transactional Analysis. I can imagine the hot potato going from one hand to the other.

Injunctions can also strongly be influenced by circumstances in which there is (temporarily) no emotional space for the child, for instance an illness or death nearby. I will illustrate the various injunctions using illustrations.

1   Don't exist
Her mother was only 16 and her father had just turned 17 when Annette was born. Her mother didn't want the child, but getting an abortion was not an option in those days. At first her parents decided to give her up for adoption. But after her father had spent a short time with her, he eventually convinced her mother to keep Annette. They would get through the tough times together. However, after two years her parents split up and against her own will, her mother was left alone with Annette.

2   Don't be you
Geraldine was born two years after her sister had died of meningitis. Her sister had also been named Geraldine.

3   Don't grow up
Peter's mother had to wait a long time before having him. She was 41 when he was conceived through IVF. Her long desire to have a baby came to pass. She would like to prevent him from getting older so he will stay with her.

4   Don't be a child
Josh was the eldest of three children. He was four years old when his father died. As from then he was 'the man of the household'.

5   Don't do anything
Patricia's mother is overprotective. She does everything for her. She dresses her, brushes her teeth and makes her sandwiches. Patricia has to sit on the back of her mother's bicycle with a helmet to school. Patricia is six years old.

6   Don't be important
Ben's younger brother Sean was handicapped. Sean always needed a lot of care from his parents. All their attention was given to Sean.

7   Don't belong
Frank's parents were expats. During childhood he moved eight times to different places. There was hardly time for him to make friends in between. Eventually he didn't even bother.

8   Don't be close
Gemma grew up without intimacy. Her parents never touched each other and they hardly touched her. Gemma can barely remember her parents ever speaking to each other.

9   Don't feel

Karin was a great volleyball player until she got leukaemia. She survived, but she feels bad. She has put on a lot of weight and her bones are always aching. People around her tell her that she shouldn't complain and that she should be grateful for being alive.

10   Don't think

Gus had thousands of questions about life. Why are the clouds white and why is the sky blue? Why is the grass green? What happens when you die? His mother and father consistently answered: 'Don't be so difficult, son.' Gus stopped asking questions.

11   Don't be well/sane

Ellen had the usual childhood ailments although nothing serious. However, her mother kept her home from school regularly. 'Best you stay home today.' Her mother didn't think it wise to let her go on school outings because of what she regarded as Ellen's fragility.

12   Don't make it

Bert came home full of enthusiasm with his school assignment in his hands. He placed it on his father's desk, hoping his father would read it. Two days later he found his assignment in his room. His father had marked the mistakes with a red pen. Nothing was ever said about the assignment.

As mentioned before, it is the child who decides what to do with the injunction. He can give it a lot of weight or just simply ignore it. He can take it literally or transform it into something positive or all kinds of possibilities in between. The child filters out what he wants to keep out.

Assignment

> **What injunctions can you recall from your own childhood?**
> **What words would you give to them?**
> **Who specifically gave you these injunctions? And how are you still affected by them?**

What the injunctions have in common is that, within, they all bear an impossible assignment. The child exists and grows up. So children find solutions for how to deal with these injunctions. They are incredibly good at discovering ways that allow them 'to be' or to exist conditionally. 'I am allowed to exist, if…' This brings us to what is called driver messages or counterinjunctions.

Driver Messages

The driver messages offer us a kind of escape clause. The child looks for the conditions under which he is allowed to exist, to be close, et cetera. He learns to specify behaviour which he believes will gain his parent's approval or at least won't be disapproved of. The child will then show this behaviour and be rewarded for it.

Ingrid's father couldn't stand it when she contradicted him. 'You have no say in this house', he would yell. 'The only thing you have to do is listen' (injunction" don't be yourself / don't be important). In the evening she would often stand behind her father's chair and start to massage his neck and shoulders with her tiny hands. He would then mutter softly: 'That's the way I like you, daddy's little princess.' This is how Ingrid came to the conclusion that she was only appreciated by her father if she pleased him. She decided not to go against her father anymore, but to subordinate herself to him and to take care of him.

The child then turns the driver messages (from the Parent) into driver behaviour. By doing this the child will receive approval from the parent. The child puts on a mask in order to be accepted by the parent. This driver behaviour will protect the child (and at a later stage the grown-up) from (temporarily) feeling the injunction.

The driver messages can be classified into five or six kinds of messages. I will describe all six messages because the last message (which is often not mentioned in TA books) is very important.

1   Be Strong

You are allowed 'to be' if you are strong, you carry all the weight and make your own decisions, so you won't be a burden to us. In your behaviour it is noticeable that you are capable of managing your own affairs and you find it difficult to accept support from others; both in a practical and an emotional sense. People with this driver often talk about themselves in terms of 'you'. By doing so, they literally disassociate themselves from their own being and inner world.

Gerald didn't take a single day off of work after both his parents had died in a short space of time. 'You just simply have to move on', he said. 'You can't let inertia win the day, that won't get you anywhere.' Thereafter he basically never spoke to anyone about it.

2   Hurry Up

You are allowed 'to be' if you get on with it and get a lot of work done in a short time, so nobody will ever have to wait for you. In their way of being, Hurry Up people usually work hard and fast and also move at a fast pace. That doesn't mean to say that this behaviour is in correspondence with their own personal experience. In fact, they have a tendency to work and move fast because they think of themselves as (too) slow.

The director was quick in everything. He talked fast, walked fast and jumped from one thing to the next. Walking next to him in the hallway I almost had to run to keep up, whilst he was talking and waving his arms around in the air.

3   Try Hard

You are allowed 'to be' if you do your best and you make and show your willingness to take on all kinds of tasks. Showing your enthusiasm is much more important than achieving success. People with a Try Hard driver often take on new projects enthusiastically and can easily leave the job unfinished because something else has come to their attention. They often have a lot of things scattered around on their desk and they always create a certain amount of chaos around them. They have difficulty sorting things out and structuring them.

Aisha is always at the front of the row when a new project comes around. Because she takes on tasks so easily, she is always drowning in work. Recently her supervisor told her to stop taking on more work and finish what she has started.

4   Please People

You are allowed 'to be' if you continuously please others. People with a Please People driver go out of their way to please others whatever the cost; to ensure that others are sitting comfortably, are getting something nice to eat and that they feel at ease. Focussing on others is often at their own expense because by doing this they (emotionally) undermine themselves.

She can't sit still for one minute at the party. She runs around offering the guests all kinds of snacks and insists they eat. When somebody says 'no' to one of the snacks, within seconds she gets back to him with something else.

5   Be Perfect

You are allowed 'to be' if you do everything perfectly. Be Perfect people want to do everything to perfection. Only an A is good enough. They are extremely well-organised, accurate and punctual. They are often well-dressed, although not necessarily. Sometimes they care less about their appearance and more about internally structuring their thoughts in a logical and precise way.

Kevin is having trouble finishing off his article. He keeps on finding new information that he would like to use. The deadline for him to submit the article has been exceeded twice and he has used three times the number of words that is permitted.

6   Be the best

You are allowed 'to be' if you are the best. In this case it is not about perfectionism, but about being better than others. Be the best people are often competitive and constantly compare themselves to others. They are out there to win.

Andrew sees everything as a competition. At work he wants to achieve the highest turnover, when cycling he always wants to be the first to arrive and he even begrudges his five-year old daughter a win at a game of cards.

Most people recognise two or three drivers they are initially triggered into the moment they are under pressure.

People often enjoy working well, pleasing others, working accurately, et cetera. Driver behaviour occurs as a reaction to stress and is unhelpful and often harmful to oneself. When in driver behaviour you are dealing with internal stress arising from injunctions you experienced as a child.

When Frank, son of expats, enters a new work environment he always immediately feels like an outsider. Everybody knows each other and he is a stranger amongst them. In response he works very hard in order to show everyone that he is the best at what he does.

When a child shows driver behaviour,

they are seeking approval from their parents.

Assignment

Think of a situation when you were under pressure.

> **What driver behaviour do you tend to perform?**
> **How do you act? What do you do?**
> **What kind of behaviour can others observe?**
> **Are you able to recognise the underlying injunction that is causing this behaviour?**

In which way does your life resemble your parents' life?

Regularly I am asked whether certain injunctions are linked to certain driver behaviour. The answer is 'no'. Although some connections may seem obvious (for example 'Don't feel' and 'Be Strong'), it is always the child who 'investigates and discovers' the kinds of behaviour that will lead to acceptance.

Program

The last component of script to be described is the program. This aspect of script consists of the ways we learn to behave in order to carry out our script. At a young age we copy our parents' program. We learn from the way they lead their lives: the relationships we enter into, the work (environment) we choose, how we maintain family relationships, how we raise our children.

We can't always determine the circumstances of our lives. But we can decide how to respond to these circumstances. Our reaction to events and situations is often driven by a profound loyalty towards (the behavioural pattern of) our parents. We often copy the behavioural pattern of the same-sex parent.

Carol's father was an alcoholic. She loathed him when he was drunk. He used to yell and become violent towards her mother. She hated seeing her mother let him treat her like that. Thirty years later Carol was living with an alcoholic, which she never would have believed possible as a child.

Reciprocity?

Many of us experience on a daily basis how parents and children mutually influence each other. The creation of script isn't just a one-way street in which the parent alone is transmitting and the child is merely receiving. Children also give their parents messages about 'who' and 'what' they are in this life by the way in which they ask for attention and relate. They thereby sometimes confirm 'old' patterns and also, regularly, new paths are opened.

For a long time Annette, who was initially going to be put up for adoption by her young parents, didn't want to have a child. She decided differently when at thirty she met a man with whom she wanted to share her life. From the first moment she held her daughter Karin in her arms, she felt it was right. She welcomed Karin into the world unconditionally and Annette too felt unconditionally welcome in the world.

Again and again our resilience and our desire for growth and development enables us to reconnect.

Intermezo

In the course of the Leadership Development Program, Carl, the man in the prologue who had lost his son, made some important discoveries about his script. He found out that, apart from not speaking about his son's death to anyone, there were many other episodes in his life that he had hidden away from others and himself. He also discovered that he was decreasingly sharing things with his life partner, which came from his belief that eventually you have to 'bear the weight alone'.

Carl knows this pattern very well. 'It is what I've been spoon-fed since I was little', he tells me at some point. 'You have to look after yourself, no one else will do it for you. That's how our father drilled us whenever we were afraid or when we didn't know what to do. He just walked away and let us stand there.' In answer to my question if he knew anything about his father's past, Carl tells me the story he remembers. 'My father never knew his father. He had left his mother before he was born. His mother was always feeling either ill or poorly. At a very young age he had to take care of things by himself. And that is what he did. After finishing engineering school he got a job, got married, had three children and always worked hard to make ends meet. There was very little tenderness at home. My parents didn't share much with each other. They hardly had any friends, only some relatives from my mother's side of the family. My father often yelled at us and sometimes he hit us. I made sure I had my tasks done to perfection.'

When we take a closer look at the script messages, Carl immediately recognises a number of messages:

Injunctions

Don't be close
Don't feel
Don't be a child

Drivers

Be Strong
Be Perfect

Carl needed some time to recognise the permissions. After a while he says: 'My father wanted us to have success. When we achieved something he was always very proud of us, all three of us. And all three of us have done well in life. We can all support ourselves. He certainly took care of that with his demanding behaviour.

We continue to explore a little further: 'Did he do it out of love?' I ask Carl.

C: *(after a long silence)... All in all I think he did. He was trying to do what he thought best for us. He didn't want us to have a life like his. He genuinely meant it. But it was tough, so tough. ...(tears come rolling down his cheeks)*

LK: *That was painful for you.*

*C:	...(sniffs) Indescribable*
*LK:	Thank you for sharing this.*

By getting in touch with his pain and sadness about his childhood, Carl takes a second important step in order to get in touch with his own being. At the same time he is having a new experience. He is allowed to show his sadness and he is given support. These are healing experiences, which should not be underestimated. They provide a starting point for Carl to learn that he is able to relate to himself and the world around him in a different way. He may remove the mask of power and perfection so he can gradually allow himself to share more, be more vulnerable and feel more.

Our resilience and our desire for growth and

development enables us to reconnect.

Fourth Act:
How the Script is developed

8. Strokes

They do not love that do not show their love.

William Shakespeare, 'The Two Gentlemen of Verona', Act 1, Scene 2

In the previous chapters I described how people develop a life script. In the following two chapters I will touch more deeply on how, in contact with others, script decisions are arrived at and how we then make our choices. I will start explaining the concept of strokes, followed by the meaning of emotions in relation to the development of script.

An important motor for script decisions is our need for recognition. In Transactional Analysis this is defined by the word stroke. In this chapter I will answer the following questions:

what are strokes
what are the different types of strokes
how we deal with strokes in our lives
how do we structure our time

The word stroke as used in TA has been derived from the verb *to stroke*, which can mean either 'caress' or 'slap'. The definition of stroke in TA is: a unit of recognition, either positive or negative.

Types of Strokes
Four types of strokes are distinguished:

1.   **Positive conditional:** the positive strokes you get for doing something. For instance, the teacher saying to the pupil 'You have written a really good essay John' or a manager saying to his employee 'You have prepared a substantial report Carla'.
2.   **Positive unconditional:** the positive strokes you get for who you are. Like a mother saying to her child 'It is always lovely when you are here' or the husband telling his wife 'Every day I'm happy with you, just the way you are'.

3. **Negative conditional**: the negative strokes you get for doing something. For instance, a father telling his son 'You make such a mess of your bedroom' or one colleague telling the other colleague 'You're such a slow worker, we'll never finish the job in time'.

4. **Negative unconditional**: the negative strokes you get for who you are. Like a mother saying to her daughter 'The day you were born was the worst day of my life' or a manager telling his employee 'You started here as a nobody and you'll leave as a nobody'.

These strokes can be given both verbally or non-verbally. We give strokes all day long. Almost every interaction between people contains an element of either a positive or a negative value judgment, in spoken words or gestures.

Assignment

> **What type of positive stroke have you received lately? Who gave it to you? What impact did it have on you?**
> **What type of positive stroke have you given recently? To whom did you give it? What was the effect?**
> **What type of negative stroke have you received lately? Who gave it to you? What impact did it have on you?**
> **What type of negative stroke have you given lately? To whom? What effect did that have on the other person?**

It goes without saying that positive strokes are the most pleasurable and nurturing. It is however necessary to add some significant comments to this statement.

How Do We Deal With Strokes in Our Lives?

To illustrate how people deal with strokes I will use a traffic metaphor: strokes are the fuel of our lives. People (and animals) need some form of touch in order to develop. By nature we develop at our best on the basis of positive strokes: conditional, unconditional, verbal, non-verbal. But at the same time, now and again, conditional negative strokes are also necessary in order to teach respect for boundaries.

At a very young age we figure out how to behave in the pursuit of 'earning' positive strokes. We tend to repeat this behaviour over and over again for the sake of receiving a 'reward'.

> *'You've helped me so magnificently with the cooking John. I just love it when we're in the kitchen together preparing meals.'*
> *'You really are good at tidying up your room.'*

Strokes are not always shared out richly. That has a lot to do with the culture in which we have been raised. It is sometimes as if it were a 'rare commodity'. That is why Claude Steiner, one of the earliest Transactional Analysts, called it 'the stroke economy'. He says that people deal with the exchange of strokes, both giving and receiving, as if they are like money within an economy. We do this according to the myth that there is a stroke shortage and that you therefore:

Do not give strokes, even if someone has earned them.
Gerald has been managing the project fantastically for the past year. Nobody has yet told him how well he is doing.

Do not ask for strokes, even if you would like them.
Although he often wonders about it, he daren't ask his supervisor whether she is satisfied with his work.

Do not accept a stroke, even if you want it.
When a colleague eventually tells him that he has done a good job, he mumbles: 'It's not such a big deal. I'm just doing my job'.

Do not reject a stroke, even though you don't want it.
A week later his supervisor goes to Gerald and tells him that she had noticed some linguistic errors in his final report. She says nothing about the contents. Gerald answers by saying that he will pay more attention the next time and he thanks his supervisor for her feedback. He can learn from it, he says.

Do not give yourself strokes
Without giving himself any kind of reward, Gerald re-engages into the next project.

Assignment

What type of strokes are easy for you to receive? What types are harder to receive?
What type of strokes are easy for you to give? What types are harder for you to give?
Which stroke economy 'rules' do you recognise with regard to yourself?
And with regard to your environment: at work and in your private life?

Stroke Economy

From our own experiences, we build our so-called stroke economy. We decide for ourselves how we deal with giving and receiving strokes. We learn to filter or shut out those strokes that don't match our self-image and to pick out those that do match the way we see ourselves. In Gerald's case, he finds it hard to accept the positive stroke, despite his desire for one; instead he gives full attention to the negative strokes. He 'thrives' in a cold stroke climate.

Regularly I came across teams with the desire to learn how to give feedback. When I inquire a bit further it always seems to be about the ability to give each other wholehearted critique. Together we then uncover the underlying conviction that they think that 'negative feedback (criticism) is what we can really learn from!

I now invite you to picture the above-mentioned economic metaphor in your mind and follow the process. We long for recognition. If this recognition is a 'rare commodity' then we go out seeking for situations in which we can get this recognition in the form of strokes. We then, on that basis, organise our lives and structure our time.

Time Structuring

Eric Berne identified a number of ways in which we structure our time. He called this time structuring. By structuring our time we meet our need for structure. Within this structure we ensure that we get the strokes we desire.

The kind of strokes you get depend on the way you structure your time and this can vary. When you withdraw, you will have to make do with the strokes you give to yourself. However, a genuinely close encounter with another person may bring you many strokes.

In the course of our upbringing we develop different forms of time structuring. In the process, the child pays close attention to the way his parents and society structure time within the entire social system.

Bob is very active in the voluntary sector, just like his father. His wife Renee, however, prefers to stay at home and read. That's how things used to be at her parent's house.

When, in the environment you grew up in, it was customary to connect with others and yourself, it will feel safe for you to do this. But if you grew up in an environment where people were afraid of closeness or even felt threatened by it, it won't be easy for you to have close relationships later on in life. As a result you may get fewer strokes from others, although you may still get more strokes from others than you give yourself.

I will begin to describe the forms of time structuring in which the social risk in relation to others (the risk of being rejected by others) is low as well as the stroke yield. I will then move towards the form of time structuring in which you take more social risk in relation to others, resulting in a higher stroke yield.

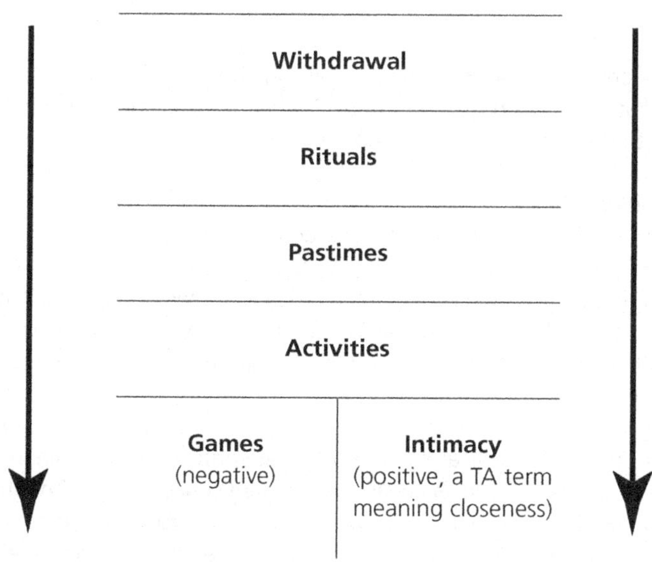

Withdrawal

When you withdraw, you distance yourself either physically or emotionally in relation to the other (or to yourself). By doing so you avoid the stokes (positive or negative) you could be receiving. It could however be that by withdrawing, you experience many internal strokes. By seeking silence and time alone or closing yourself off from stimuli, you are actually taking care of yourself. Withdrawing now and again gives you the opportunity to restore the balance and to recharge your batteries in between experiences and contact with people.

> Hank was often bullied when he was a child. Outside of work he doesn't really talk to anyone. He prefers to be on his own.
> Anna loves to socialise, but now and again she has a need to withdraw. Otherwise she gets over-excited by all the impressions and interactions with people and, in her words, she 'flips out'.

Rituals

Rituals consist of a familiar and predictable interaction between people.

> They had been together for years. She cooks, he lays the table. They eat their meal in silence after which she makes coffee and he does the dishes. He then goes to watch TV.
> When they meet, their conversation always follows the same pattern. They tell each other about work and how their children are. After a while they get out the backgammon board and play a couple of games.

Pastimes

Picture people together chatting about one or two topics without an aim or objective. Pastimes are often used to gauge the other person before entering into more significant, closer contact.

> At the party I end up in 'the men's corner' talking about football and cars.
> On the first date with her boyfriend she talks about the weather and how hot and dry it has been this Spring. He chats along eagerly.

Activities (work and/or hobby)

The interaction or contact is aimed at achieving a goal.

> A number of times a year we clean up the garden together to keep it looking nice.
> In their circle of friends they always help each other out when someone is moving house. They tease each other a bit, but they also give each other compliments.

Games

This kind of game is a psychological game, not to be confused with ordinary games children and grown-ups play for fun. Game is an important concept within TA. Therefore I will go into it in more detail in Chapter 13. What is necessary to know for now is that, when interacting, a game initially involves an ulterior motive and it will often result in a predictable negative outcome for at least one, but usually for all players of the game. In this pattern of interaction it is possible to 'earn' a lot of negative strokes. Ultimately this is all about contact that appears to be intimate, a 'seeming intimacy', but it is actually not.

Geraldine often grumbles at herself because of the mess Hugh makes. She always cleans up after him. He gets furious because he doesn't want her to put her hands on his stuff. She then starts to cry and after some hesitation he puts his arm around her and comforts her.

Intimacy

This contact involves expressing feelings and needs to each other in a genuine way. Persons involved have a high level of awareness, spontaneity and openness. Within this form of time structuring both the investment risk (maximum vulnerability) as well as the possible stroke yield are the highest.

They face one another in silence. They look into each other's eyes and she carefully takes his hand. She has hurt his feelings and he is angry. He asks her not to do it again. She tells him that she sincerely regrets what she has said and she apologises. They look at each other and eventually nod when they feel that they are OK again.

It probably hardly needs saying that the dividing line between the various forms of time structuring isn't as clear as I have drawn above. They often overlap with one another.

Assignment

Take a look at your own time structuring in the past week.

> **How much time do you spend on each form of time structuring?**
> **Does it provide you with a lot of strokes?**
> **What kind of strokes do you get?**
> **Is this to your satisfaction?**

How could you increase the yield? What would you have to do / stop doing to achieve that? And what about the other(s)?

In conclusion

People can't do without strokes. They prefer to receive negative strokes rather than have none at all. This kind of thinking has far-reaching implications for the way our education system and organisations are managed.

At school, Patrick never got told if he had done well. At a certain point he was considered remedial. He started to tease his classmates and his teachers. That's how he could always be assured of getting a sufficient amount of strokes.

Management of a pharmaceutical company strived for perfection. The monitoring of the process consisted of an extreme number of checks and balances. Excellent performance was the norm. When mistakes were made, managers would have a performance review for at least half an hour. Nevertheless, employees kept on making a lot of mistakes. Not really surprising considering that this was the only way to have direct contact with your boss.

People prefer to receive negative strokes

rather than none at all.

9. Emotions

Give sorrow words. The grief that does not speak whispers the

o'er-fraught heart, and bids it break.

William Shakespeare, 'Macbeth', Act 4, Scene 3

The way you deal with your emotions is of particular importance with regard to the way you develop your life script. In this chapter I will elaborate on:

the significance of emotions
emotions and script
rackets

The Significance of Emotions

TA recognises four authentic or primary human emotions: Fear, Anger, Happiness and Sadness. These emotions all, in their own way, have a physical impact. There are of course other emotions that can be distinguished, but these are mixtures of the four primary emotions. You could compare it with the way we look at colours; red, blue and yellow being the primary colours.

Each emotion has its own significance. The emotion sets either yourself and/or your environment in motion. An event occurs triggering a need. Subsequently an emotion arises upon which we act in order to respond adequately to the event.

The sequence is as follows:

Event   Need   Feeling   Behaviour   Satisfaction of need (peace)

According to John Parr, an English psychotherapist, our primary emotion is one of happiness, varying from satisfied to cheerful.

When a disturbing event occurs, the other emotions pop up in order to help us return to the peaceful state of happiness.

Our emotions stem from parts of the brain that are not easy for us to consciously control. They're like reflexes that are set into motion when certain events occur.

I will now walk you through the four primary emotions and their significance.

Fear

The feeling of fear brings you in contact with your need for safety. On the basis of this emotion you can be prompted into three kinds of actions: fight, flight or freeze. Each of these actions can be an adequate response to a certain situation.

> *A boy approaches me in a threatening manner. I stand firm, make eye contact and push him away.*
> *People start a riot at the market square. I make a run for it.*
> *A barking dog is running towards me. I stand still, continue to breath peacefully and avoid eye contact.*

Authentic fear is always about something that is going to happen in the (near) future.

Assignment

> **Can you recall the last time you felt fear?**
> **What caused you to feel fearful?**
> **What was your need at the time?**
> **What did you do?**
> **What was the effect?**

Anger

The feeling of anger brings you in contact with your need for boundaries. On the basis of this emotion you are prompted to either set, watch over or restore your boundaries.

> *Somebody steps on my toes. I say 'ouch' and push her away.*
> *I am being insulted by someone. I confront him and tell him that I don't want to be treated that way.*

Authentic anger is always related to something that is happening in the present.

Assignment

> **Can you recall the last time you were angry?**
> **What caused you to be angry?**
> **What was your need at the time?**
> **What did you do?**
> **What was the effect?**

Sadness

The feeling of sadness brings you in contact with your need for support. This emotion prompts you to find support from others and in return others are prompted to give you this support.

> *Andrea is curled up on the coach. She is very sad and she is sobbing. Tears are trickling down her cheeks. Her mother sits down next to her and wraps her arms around her in silence.*

Authentic sadness is always about something that has happened in the (recent) past.

Assignment

Can you recall the last time you were sad?
What caused you to be sad?
What was your need at the time?
What did you do?
What was the effect?

Happiness

The feeling of happiness brings you in contact with your need to be with others and to share. This emotion prompts you and others to connect.

At last Frank got the promotion he had been waiting for. He's really happy about that and he decides to look up some friends and share the news.
I'm sitting in a café and hear the people at the table next to me laughing out loud. I notice that I'm smiling and feel the urge to join them.

Assignment

Can you recall the last time you felt happy?
What caused you to feel happy?
What was your need at the time?
What did you do?
What was the effect?

People have a great ability to empathise with others. Recent neurological research gives us a better understanding of how the neurons in our brain 'wire and fire' together and how that gives us the ability to relate to similar (emotional) experiences upon which we respond.

Emotions and Script

The emotions described and illustrated above occur in this way by nature. However, in the course of our lives we experience disturbing situations and we learn that in certain circumstances it is better not to express certain emotions. In these situations expressions of the authentic emotions have been discouraged and in effect they are either suppressed or get substituted by inauthentic emotions. Neurological pathways get shut off, whilst others are opened up instead.

Steven could never get angry. Even if people made his life a misery, he would always keep on smiling. In one of our coaching sessions he tells me that nobody ever quarrelled or got into a fight at his parental home. As an only child he grew up in a harmonious household in which he and his parents were always nice to each other.

Frank was born and raised as the son of a farmer. 'Let's make it happen' was the motto. Feelings of sadness were for wimps. After his wife passed away, Frank could only feel anger. He was very angry.

Assignment

Which of the primary emotions do you find hard to access?

It gets confusing when you experience emotions that are actually substituting your authentic emotions. In general this leads to undesirable outcomes. In Steven's case, he is at risk that people take even more advantage of him because he is not clear about his boundaries. He invites them to do so with his smile. And Frank possibly keeps people at a distance with his anger, although deep down inside he wants to be comforted. We often find it hard to get in touch with our authentic needs. Steven's smile is almost stuck on his face. It's the mask through which he has learned to view the world.

That's how we, mostly out of awareness, create outcomes we haven't intended, whilst at the same time these outcomes reinforce our perception of the world.

Assignment

> **Which of your emotions emerges easily?**
> **Is this emotion always appropriate, given the situation? (Explore whether the nature of the emotion fits the following situations: fear – future; angry – present; sad – past)**
> **What is the outcome? Does this emotion get you what you want?**

Rackets

Emotions that are not in sync with the situation are called *racket feelings* in TA. In English a racket is defined as: 'the money you pay to a person in order to protect you or your belongings from that same person'. Think of how gangsters operate. That's all about extortion money. And that's exactly how racket feelings work in the sense that they extort others.

Whenever somebody got angry with Carla she would always start to cry. Mostly the other person then stops being angry and will start to comfort her by saying things such as "I didn't mean it like that' and 'It's alright, calm down'. This had become a habit for Carla, even when there was reason for her to be angry herself. When I ask her whether she ever got angry, she immediately replies: 'No, never.'

The authentic feeling gets pushed away by a more familiar feeling that then replaces the authentic feeling. This replacement of feelings is done out of awareness. This so-called substitution of feelings and the behaviour that goes with it is a learned behaviour as a way of earning strokes in childhood. We therefore continuously repeat the behaviour. The racket feeling eventually becomes our 'favourite bad feeling'. The authentic, underlying need, however, is not being met and the inner restlessness continues to exist.

When I asked Carla what she would like, after thinking about it for quite some time, she decided that she wanted to be taken seriously and that others would let her stand on her own two feet. When I commented that this would be difficult for her to achieve because she is so used to 'having an arm around her', she started to cry.

Even though the behaviour is ineffective, it gets repeated over and over again in the hope that our needs will eventually be met. This repetition results in the reinforcement of the script.

Carla looked up after she noticed that I wasn't responding to her tears. She sat up straight and looked at me. 'And now what?', she asked.

The sequence is as follows:

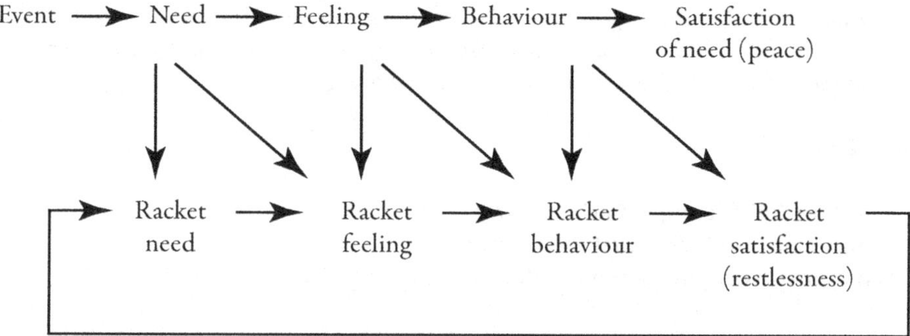

Racket Behaviour
In childhood we often learn not to show certain emotions, but we substitute them with racket feelings. The behaviour that we then show is actually a strategy we have learned at an earlier stage in life in order to (temporarily) have our needs met.

The sequence is as follows:

Racket behaviour has a manipulative quality towards others, although we don't always manipulate others. We often manipulate ourselves.

When Gerald feels helpless at work, he always goes out for a run. He runs at least five times a week. He never resolves the conflict at work.

When Caroline is at home alone, she empties the entire biscuit tin.

In view of this process people have often completely lost touch with their underlying feelings. All that remains is a poignant need that never gets satisfied.

Working with Rackets
Rackets are part of the script pattern. In advance of the next chapter, I will explain a bit about how you can already get started on finding out about your own rackets, discovering that you're dealing with inauthentic feelings and behaviour and that this behaviour will not satisfy your underlying needs.

Explore what significance rackets have for you. It will be easier to let go of racket feelings and racket behaviour once you are aware of their significance and you learn to value them as 'the best choice you could have made in the past'.

Decide on the emotion and kind of behaviour you would like to develop and determine what this could provide you with. Seek out situations in which you can experiment. Practice, practice, practice and celebrate your successes.

Carla slowly comes to understand how her sadness and fear have been like a lifeboat for her in the past. 'In a household with four boys and a tyrannical father, it was impossible for me to set my own boundaries. The only thing that helped me then were my tears. She realises that she is at risk of staying the little girl she always was. She no longer wants that. 'I want to be taken seriously at work. That's why I want to become firmer and stronger.'

Assignment

Which racket feeling is Carla dealing with?
Which emotion is she pushing away?
What positive significance did the racket feeling used to have for her?

She starts to practise this new way of feeling and behaving. Firstly, at home with her boyfriend and after a while gradually within her circle of friends. One day she proudly tells me how she had stood up to her boss. When I asked her what the outcome had been she answered: 'He was startled, and so was I. And after a while he agreed with me and apologised and then we both started to laugh.'

Assignment

Which racket feelings can you identify (well) with?
And what kind of racket behaviour do you recognise in yourself?
In what kind of situations does it arise?
Where did you learn to do this?
Which significance did this have for you?
What is the underlying authentic need?
What kind of behaviour would meet that need?
What is holding you back?

Intermezzo

Caroline, the cheerful young lady mentioned in the prologue, gets emotional when we talk about the way she is fulfilling her life. 'In my environment it's all about keeping up appearances. We're all busy doing our houses up, going out for meals and showing each other how well we're doing. It's very superficial and I simply go along with it.' When I ask her what is making her go along with things, she replies: 'I have never learned any differently. This is what I know. I told you before that things were good at home when I was growing up. But the focus was all on the outside, the whole respectable white-picket fence family thing. My parents wanted us to have all our material needs met and for us to be happy. They went out of their way for us. We never had any deep and meaningful conversations.'

I then give her an outline of the different forms of time structuring, varying from withdrawal to intimacy, and I ask her to think of the way she fills in her time. It doesn't take her long to answer: 'Mostly pastimes and activities', she says without a doubt. 'It is all very superficial.' In our next session together I explain the concept of 'script' to her and ask her what she used to do in order to get strokes:

C: *By being a cheerful and friendly girl*
LK: *You did that well?*
C: *Absolutely*
LK: *What happened whenever you got angry or sad?*
C: *Nothing*
LK: *What do you mean by 'nothing'?*
C: *Exactly what I said: 'Nothing'. My parents and my brothers ignored me. So I didn't show these feelings to them. I used to shut myself in my room.*
LK: *And what do you do now you're older?*
C: *(thoughtful) The same, I think. My boyfriend isn't comfortable with emotions and I give my sadness and anger a wide berth. (silence). I've been feeling quite dissatisfied and resentful lately, but I'm holding it inside me.*
LK: *It seems to me that you're paying a high price for a 'happy life'.*
C: *Yes I am.*

I explain the meaning of the various emotions to Caroline and we talk about racket feelings. With a sigh of relief she claims that she is not allowed to have feelings of sadness and anger and that in all cases the racket feeling is 'Happy'. I ask her what her relief is about. She replies: 'I've always known deep down inside that something wasn't right. Now I'm starting to understand.' And then she goes on to say decisively: 'How are we going to tackle this?' Her first assignment is to share her insights with her partner. I also ask her to keep track of her emotions during the next two weeks by journaling the emotions she feels in relation to the situations she is in and to determine whether or not her emotions are authentic.

For Caroline these first steps are important. To be able to get in touch with her passion, she will have to learn to distinguish and feel her emotions. In addition it is also important that she involves people in her current social environment in her personal growth. They, after all, play an important part with regard to her behavioural development.

10. Working with your script patterns

If to do were as easy as to know what were good to do, chapels

had been churches and poor men's cottages princes' palaces.

William Shakespeare, 'The Merchant of Venice' Act 1, Scene 2

In the previous chapter I elaborated on the creation of script patterns. This chapter is about the possibility to change undesirable script patterns. To stay with the metaphor of masks and cosmetics we will seek to answer the question 'how to remove the make-up'.

Striving for Autonomy

Your script restricts your autonomy. You act on the basis of old habits, not being able to look openly at what is actually happening and whether your usual reactions give an adequate response to the situation.

Autonomy is the ability to act in response to the here-and-now reality. We then no longer let ourselves be guided by old messages and experiences, but are able to look at what is happening in the moment. The following four terms are closely connected with autonomy.

Awareness – of yourself, others and your environment. Awareness is about your ability to live in the here-and-now and to experience things as they present themselves. You can choose to see, feel and smell life in all its colours instead of chasing yourself trying to live up to the demands of society and your own expectations.

One day Eddy decides to sell his successful business. He had gotten tired of running around not knowing in which direction he was heading. He wanted to live a more meaningful life for himself and the world around him. He took a part time job at a school to teach technical engineering and looked after his children twice a week. Although he has taken a step down with regard to his financial and societal status, he is enjoying every minute of his life.

Intimacy – This is about your ability to be in an open relationship with others. You are capable of sharing your needs and desires openly with others and you have the ability to interact lovingly with other people.

Karin and Astrid have been friends for a very long time. In their friendship they have a lot of fun, but they can also quarrel, have great conversations and be silent. They both have complete trust in each other.

Spontaneity – This relates to your ability to react genuinely and without inhibitions in the moment. It's about being able to experience and show authentic feelings such as fear, anger, happiness and sadness and other mixed feelings that go with them. According to Berne, founder of Transactional Analysis, this is about liberation; being liberated by showing feelings even if they were not learned as permitted in childhood.

She expresses her first words of anger with hesitance. She looks at me with a pleading look on her face. 'Go on, it's alright', I say encouragingly, after which the anger floods out of her mouth. After a while she shouts out from the bottom of her heart: 'Damn it, damn it, damn it!' after which she starts shrieking with laughter, opening the path for change.

Integrity – Developing intimacy, spontaneity and awareness leads to an increased level of integrity. The meaning of integrity here is about wholeness. The more you are able to integrate your experiences into your Adult, the bigger your sense of wholeness will be.

For many years she had been working at a large number of missions in all kinds of disadvantaged areas. She had experienced a lot in her life. Now, at seventy years of age, she radiated a natural wholeness and peace.

An autonomous human being is aware of themself, others and the environment, is able to respond spontaneously, is capable of sharing intimacy with self and others and experiences themself as a whole person.

Assignment

> **Can you recall moments in which you felt autonomous in a way described above?**
> **When and where did you feel it?**
> **What were you doing?**
> **What were you thinking?**
> **What were you feeling?**

Redecisions

The Adult ego-state plays an important role in the course of autonomy development. Being able to respond to what is happening in the here-and-now occurs from the Adult ego-state. However, in order to get to this stage it is sometimes necessary to reconsider your decision about what and who you are in this world. Your script decisions can limit you and continue to pull you back into your old response patterns. Therefore, people working with TA often pay attention to the so-called re-decisions. The point at which one can make a re-decision is illustrated at the top of the following page using the script circle from Chapter 6.

At a young age Gus decided that he should take care of other people. He has always derived a lot of his being from helping others. He gets a lot of recognition working in health care. He recently was appointed manager. Overall he is doing a good job. But when he has to make a tough decision, for instance on the working hours of employees, he gets tensed up. He gets out of balance when employees complain about his decisions because he wants everyone to be happy.

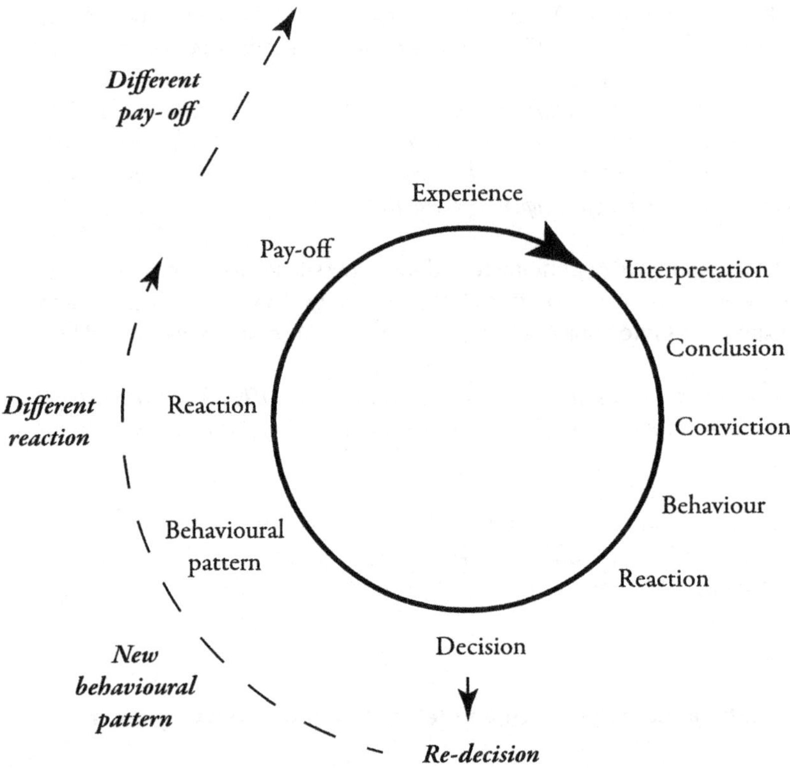

After a number of conv ersations he realises that he's on a dead end street. 'If I want to make everyone happy, I will end up having a nervous breakdown', he sighs. He then makes a very important decision: 'I am allowed to confront my employees for the sake of giving good service to our clients who, after all, we are here for.'

Gus' redecision is an important moment in his personal growth. It has opened up new horizons and new opportunities. However, a redecision by itself is not enough to change behaviour. The new habit has to be ingrained in the way his old habit with regard to 'always helping others' had been ingrained earlier. In order to learn and integrate new habits it is necessary to look back, gain new experiences and celebrate your successes.

Looking Back

To be able to let go of old behavioural patterns, it is necessary to understand and acknowledge the value this behaviour has had in your own life history. You need to do this so your own life story will remain consistent and logical. When you succeed in doing this, you will be able to let go of old patterns and learn new ones.

At a certain point Gus starts to understand why he is always focussed on caring for others. 'My father was often ill and my mother could hardly manage and at a young age I started to feel very responsible for them. And I received a lot of recognition and compliments for being helpful.

My mother used to say: 'If I hadn't had Gus around... and I remember how I radiated pride.' Gus then added: 'I know that the caring side of me is one of my main strengths and I wouldn't want to lose it. But I also feel the need to add other things in to my behavioural repertoire, without being afraid that people might not like me anymore.'

Gaining New Experiences

To develop it is necessary to gain new experiences and to notice that the new behaviour is very beneficial. Initially you often have to bite the proverbial bullet. And you also should take into account that your (social) environment will have to get used to your new behaviour and might want to pressure you not to change. In order to resist this pressure you will need a lot of determination and possibly a support system to encourage you on your journey.

Gus and I are having our last session together. We look back at the process that has taken place during the last six months. 'It was difficult in the beginning', he says. 'I knew what I wanted, namely a more efficient and effective duty roster in the department, but it was a real ordeal to resist my colleagues' tears. And it became even more difficult when some of my colleagues told me that I wasn't a good team leader. Luckily my supervisor supported me, otherwise I doubt whether I would have been able to survive.' He ends up by saying: 'It was actually just a week ago that I felt certain of myself because of the positive feedback my colleagues gave me during the yearly review. They said that I was doing a good job, not always an easy person, but firm and fair. Now I know for sure that I am on the right track.'

Celebrating Success

To conclude with, it's really nice to celebrate your successes. You could consider this to be a kind of a ritual in order to get closure on the process that you have been through. This is also an important beacon upon which you can proudly look back as well as a starting point from which you can take new steps.

I asked Gus how he was going to celebrate his success. With a big smile on his face he answered: 'This afternoon I'm going to treat myself to a sauna.'

Assignment

Go back to the script circle.

Make a plan of action for yourself using the following questions:

What is my (re-)decision?
How shall I behave?
In which situations or context?
With whom?
When am I going to do this?
How will I know that I have achieved my results?
How will I reward myself for this?

Working with Drivers and Injunctions

When you are affected by an injunction, it could be helpful to talk to somebody about it who is professionally trained: a psychotherapist or a counsellor. They can help you find your way.

Apart from getting professional help, it is very beneficial to look after yourself in daily life. You can ask others (your life partner, a close friend or maybe even your parents) for the permissions that you might not have received whilst growing up. You can also give yourself permission. Do it attentively.

Geraldine, who struggles with being close to others (and herself), sometimes asks her best friend to hold her. She also regularly goes for a massage. During the day she repeatedly says to herself 'I am allowed to make contact with others' and sometimes she says it out loud.

At some stage driver behaviour was formed in order to compensate for one or more injunctions. In order to achieve behavioural change, you usually won't get the outcome you would like if you only pay attention to your drivers. Before dealing with your driver behaviour, it will be necessary to therapeutically deal with the underlying injunctions.

Barbara has started to become aware that she doesn't constantly need to take care of others. She is trying hard to stop doing it, but that's making her feel desperate. She feels that, without being able to care for and please others, she is worthless and that she might just as well not exist. With her counsellor's help, Barbara gets to work on her self-image and self-esteem and slowly but surely she starts accepting herself for who she is, increasingly able to meet her own needs instead of putting all her energy into others.

Very often there are two sides to a coin, especially when it comes to activities that help you connect with yourself and others. Mainly physical activities are known to have a huge effect on reconnecting with oneself, which is understandable considering the fact that most injunctions stem from the time before you were able to speak as a child.

Hans' parents were always arguing. At a young age he had learned to be a sweet and kind little boy and not to be a bother to anybody. During secondary school he struggled with this behaviour. He daren't say 'no' to anyone. Luckily, Family Services gave him the opportunity to go on an Outward Bound trips into Ireland. That helped him to become stronger and more self-confident.

Lastly I would like to give some specific recommendations on how to deal with each of the drivers:

Driver	To do
Please People	Ask others to acknowledge you unconditionally (see Chapter 8 on strokes). Focus on physical activities and a physical environment such as yoga, gardening and a warm bath. Create time and space for yourself, for example, to read a book, go to the movies or go for a walk.

Be Perfect	Ask for acknowledgment for the work you are doing. Have fun and look for fun things such as watching a comedy or humorous TV-programmes. Take on an activity to relax such as mindfulness. Look for people who are dealing with the same kind of challenges that you are facing and share experiences.
Hurry Up	Seek out a safe and fast sport, either to do or to watch.
Try Hard	Ask for acknowledgment and appreciation for what you are doing. This will help you to complete tasks. Seek out safe activities that meet your need for variation.
Be Strong	Book a holiday and be mindful about where, how and with whom. Go into a retreat, meditate, paint, write poems. Enter into personal relationships.
Be the best	Ask for acknowledgement and appreciation for who you are. Look for an individual, competitive sport in which you can discharge your desire to compete. Do nice things with others and have fun.

Driver behaviour is formed in order to compensate for one or more injunctions.

Fifth Act:
Getting the show on the road

11. Windows on the world

There is nothing either good or bad, but thinking makes it so.

William Shakespeare, 'Hamlet', Act 4, Scene 3

Introduction

In previous chapters the emphasis has been on individual development: the child growing up, the choices you make in childhood about who and what you are in life, and how these choices come about. In the course of this book, the significance of individual development with regard to relationships has gradually emerged. In the following chapters the focus will be on relationships. Human beings are after all first and foremost relational beings. We enter into relationships in a way that is predictable for ourselves and for others. We tend to play a limited number of roles in our lives. In this respect we are creatures of habit. In the chapters to come we will explore this predictability on the basis of a number of concepts, like a grid that can be placed over the complex reality to help you discover recurring patterns.

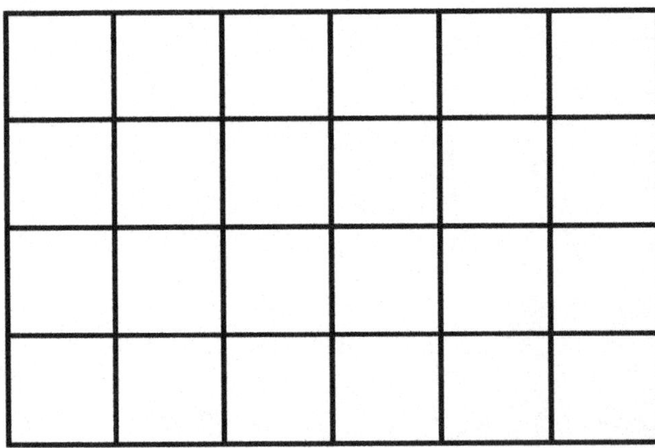

The following concepts will be discussed:

> Windows on the world
> Transference
> Games
> The drama triangle and the winner's triangle

I'm OK, You're OK

My first encounter with TA was when I found a book in one of the book cabinets in my father's study: *I'm OK, You're OK* by *Thomas A. Harris*. It was a bestseller in the seventies and still when I mention TA to people they often respond: 'Ah yes, that's about I'm OK, You're OK!' The underlying philosophy of TA and its founder, Eric Berne, was encapsulated in the title of this book. This statement reflects a belief system that each of us is OK.

Every human being is responsible for their own behaviour, including the mistakes they make. In the way we view people, we make distinctions between people by their behaviours. A person is at all times OK, even if their behaviour isn't. In previous chapters I have made clear that it is above all about the intention underlying the behaviour: what does somebody want to get out of it? This leads to the statement that 'I'm OK' and that 'You're OK'. In TA terms we call this a life position: an attitude we adopt towards others, ourselves and the world.

Assignment

Think of a recent situation in which you thought the other person's behaviour not to be OK, but you were successfully able to remain in contact.

> **What did the other person do?**
> **What did you do?**
> **How did you feel?**

In all cases in which you are able to sustain an OK-OK-position, you will be able to stay connected to the other and yourself. I highlighted this in Chapter 2 when I wrote about attachment as being the basis for healthy development.

Eric Berne also distinguished another three life positions:

> I'm OK, You're not OK.
> I'm not OK, You're not OK.
> I'm not OK, You're OK.

You can imagine that your view on yourself and the other will vary depending on the life position you adopt. You could compare it to when you're standing in front of a bay window and when looking out, depending on the window you look through, you will get a different view on the world, the so-called 'windows on the world' as illustrated below.

You're OK

I'm not OK

I'm not OK You're OK (the helpless position) - +	I'm OK You're OK (the healthy position) + +
I'm not OK You're not OK (the hopeless position) - -	I'm OK You're not OK (the arrogant position) + -

I'm OK

You're not OK

Windows on the world

Each window offers you a different view on yourself and on the world around you. In the course of our lives we all take on a certain existential life position: a view on the world that is dominant. This life position is reinforced through experience. Your window on the world is an important part of your life script. We all have a favoured life position, in which we spend most of our time. But we also step into the other windows from time to time. I will illustrate this with the following examples.

I'm OK, You're OK (the healthy position)
Existential
Maria lives according to the motto 'We give so we may receive'. She has a lot of confidence in herself and the people she is surrounded by. People can easily call upon her, as much as she seeks and accepts help whenever she is in need of it. Recently Maria launched a website in order to share all her knowledge in the legal field. Colleagues regularly send her additional information to put on her website.

A daily snapshot
Hank is in a great mood. The sun is shining and his supervisor has just given him a nice compliment. His life is wonderful and he would love to share that with the entire world.

I'm OK, You're not OK (the arrogant position)
Existential
Peter is known to be an arrogant man with an extremely sharp tongue. He is the managing director of a building company. His employees barely dare ask him anything out of fear of being ridiculed. Peter fights his way through life in the belief that 'nobody in this world of losers is

going to give you anything'. Every day he searches for mishaps in his employees' behaviours that consequently reinforce his beliefs: 'they are even too lazy to scratch their own behinds' and 'they don't deliver what they should be delivering'.

A daily snapshot
Caroline has worked hard on a project. However, chances are that they won't meet the deadline because Ernst, one of her colleagues, hasn't completed his part. For a moment she thinks: 'I should have done it myself'.

I'm not OK, You're OK (the helpless position)
Existential
Harry is always full of admiration for people around him. His wife, who is great with their kids and is also able to combine motherhood with her work as a teacher. His boss, who at such a young age has moved up the career ladder. His colleagues, who always deliver top quality work. He would never be able to compare with that. He doesn't even understand what other people see in him.

A daily snapshot
Ernst is struggling to complete his project task on time. He has great admiration for his colleague Caroline, who has it all together. 'She's probably not at all happy with me', crosses his mind before he gets back to work.

I'm not OK, You're not OK (the hopeless position)
Existential
Astrid has not been to work for weeks. She's burned out. She's had enough of herself and everyone around her. 'People are no good, especially me.' She hardly gets out of bed and she lets nobody in. The only thing she does though is chat on the internet and criticise the 'whole mess'.

A daily snapshot
Gerald is exhausted when he gets home. It hasn't been an easy day. He had gotten into an argument with one of his colleagues at work. It's a complete pandemonium in the house. The kids are tired and are crying, and his wife has burnt the roast. 'I'm not doing a good job, but they're not doing any better', he thinks and sits himself down on the couch with a big sigh.

I'm OK and You're OK.

Assignment

Imagine looking through each of the windows and think of examples from your own life that relate to each of them.

> **What happened?**
> **Where, when, with whom?**
> **What were you doing, what was the other person doing?**
> **How were you viewing yourself and the other person?**
> **Which of the life positions are you most familiar with?**
> **Out of which window have you been looking the most during the past 24 hours?**

Different Levels

You can look at your own or someone else's life position at different levels. The examples above have been described at the **social level**. This level is about how people behave in relation to the surrounding world.

It is however very likely that the life position of Peter, for example, the manager of the building company, is not the same at the psychological level. The psychological level will then be about how Peter is feeling inside.

In one of our sessions he tells me:

LK: And when you yell at that colleague of yours, how do you feel?
P: (silent) At first I feel great!
LK: And then?
P: (silent) Then I actually think I'm a bully.
LK: Could you tell me more about that?
P: (he makes a dismissive gesture) Yes well, that I'm still unable to say things in a decent way, talk things over in a decent way. When it happens, I really dislike myself.

Assignment

Take a look at your own life position examples you described earlier on, together with Peter's example. Is it recognisable? Do you ever show behaviour that is not congruent with the way you're feeling inside?

En Route To OK – OK

I often catch myself feeling either better or less than others. Both for myself and others, going through life in an OK–OK-position is, above all, an ideal to aspire to instead of an on-going stable life position.

Patrick swore that he thought of his employees as good people and that he also approached them in that manner. A few moments later the cafeteria lady passed by in the corridor pushing a rattling trolley and Patrick jumps up and groans: 'That silly woman always makes so much noise'. After he has spoken he suddenly looks at me with an embarrassed expression on his face.

It has probably become clear to you that your own script significantly influences the way you perceive others and yourself. And again, it takes a considerable amount of exercise to view things from a different perspective. Be aware to take small steps at a time and be lenient on yourself and others whilst you're taking them.

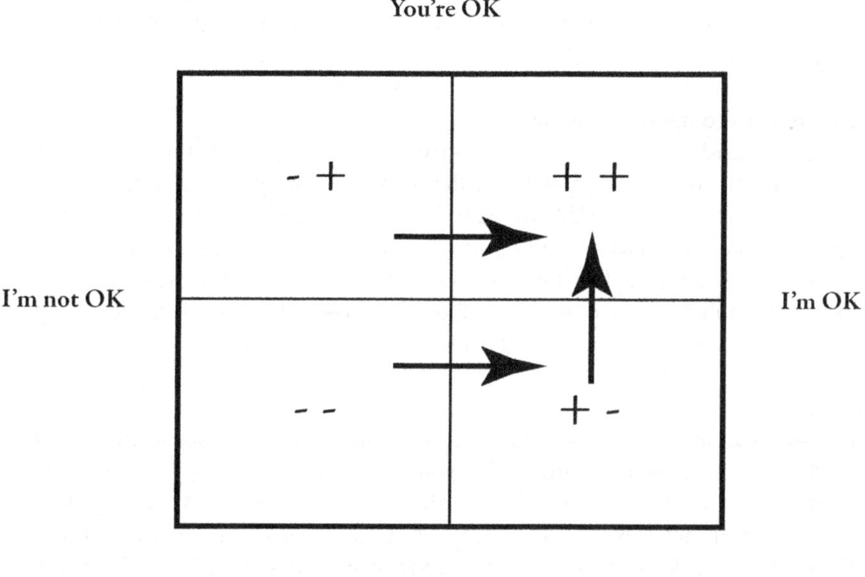

Some Practical Tips

Getting out of the - - quadrant

The biggest initial step is to increase your own self-esteem. In this respect it is important that you take good care of yourself by:

> working less
> going outside in the fresh air
> putting on a nice cologne
> taking a bath
> reading a book comfortably on the couch
> tidying up your house

Or any other way you want to take care of yourself. Give yourself permission to meet your own needs. For example; 'I am allowed to focus on myself, because I'm important.'

Progressing from - + to the + + quadrant
See the list above. Give yourself the message that you're OK just as you are and talk to others about it. Learn to value your qualities and strengths and further unleash them.

Ask for positive strokes when you need them. Be clear on what you want these strokes for. Get yourself going. Self-esteem will grow when you leave your passive attitude behind you. Create a goal or direction in life. What would you like to aim for? Make use of necessary resources. Be prepared to keep on connecting to people, even when you sometimes might tend to fall back into the - + quadrant. Stand in front of the mirror and practice how you look when you stand firmly, with a determined look in your eyes. How do you feel inside? And find a way to remind yourself to keep on doing this (tie a knot in your handkerchief).

Progressing from + - to the + + quadrant
Focus on the relationship with others. Practice expressing appreciation for others, that they will grow from. Relax yourself in a way that suits you. Avoid doing performance-oriented activities for relaxation. Have fun with yourself and others. Occasionally laugh at yourself and your own behaviour. Putting your own greatness into perspective will help you enormously. Practice your facial expressions in front of the mirror: how do I look when I make a friendly face? And how does that make me feel inside? And find a way to remind yourself to keep on doing this (tie a knot in your handkerchief).

Holding on to + +
Take good care of yourself and others. When you act, ask yourself regularly whether or not you and others are benefitting from what you are doing. Be assertive. Stand up for your own interests and have consideration for the interests of others. A confrontation can be necessary and that's OK. Pay attention to both the task you are dealing with as well as the relationship. Make sure you get enough relaxation and enjoy the moments when you're in flow.

12. Transference

Whose own hard dealings teaches them suspect the thoughts

of others!

William Shakespeare, 'The merchant of Venice', Act 1, Scene 3

In the previous chapter I shed some light on the windows on the world and how relationship patterns are repeated when you continue to position others and yourself in a certain way (+ or −).

In this chapter I will elaborate on a psychological phenomenon called 'transference'. This is not a typical TA concept. It originates from Sigmund Freud's psychoanalysis. Transference occurs when you redirect or project thoughts, feelings, needs and experiences from the past to a person in the present. In Transactional Analysis we call this 'putting a face' on to a person. This happens out of awareness.

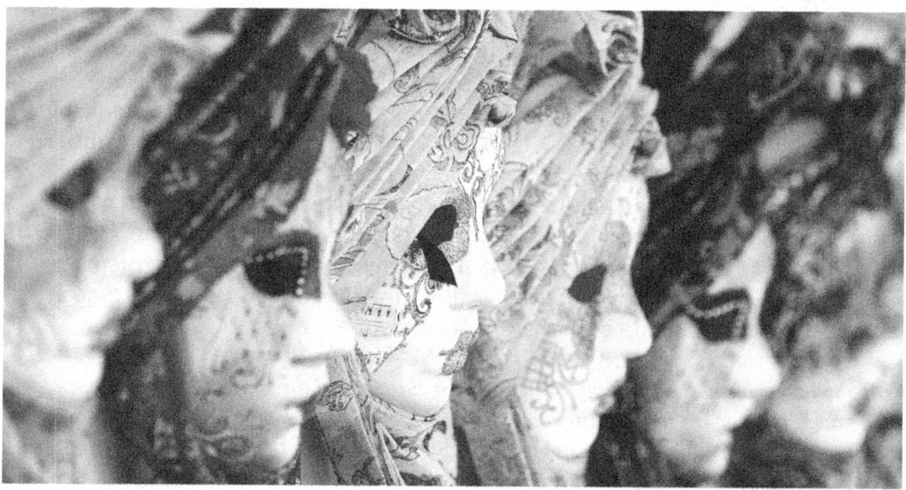

We all have our own stock of masks from the past out of which we can choose and put on to another person.

Gerald has continuing disputes with his boss. According to Gerald his boss has an authoritarian attitude, which really frustrates him. During our conv ersation on this topic I ask Gerald who his boss reminds him of. It doesn't take him long to answer: 'My father of course!'

Now being aware of this, Gerald is able to look at his boss from a different perspective and also look at himself differently, being the grown-up man that he is.

Transference plays an important part in our daily life. A lot of our behaviour is based on transference. We continuously make use of the enormous database in our bodies and search for former experiences to match each situation we encounter. It may be that our search is driven by somebody's actions, their facial expression or the way somebody smells. Your search may also be driven by the way you relate to another person, for instance an authoritarian relationship like in Gerald's case, or the environment you're in or the situation that occurs, and so forth. We call these triggers, stimuli that set something in motion.

Assignment

Think back to a recent situation in which you immediately had a negative opinion of someone without you even knowing the person. With whom did you associate this person? How come?

All in all there is a lot of 'searching' going on. Fortunately a lot of this happens out of our awareness. We make connections at lightning speed that set us in motion. In our daily lives we constantly go back and forth from present to past without being aware of or affected by it.

Brenda is 58 years old. During a group meeting, Brenda being the eldest of the group, she tells us that up till now she has had eight job interview rejections for reasons she finds hard to identify with. I then ask the other participants in the group to share the first association that Brenda triggers in each of them. The associations vary from 'wise' to 'strict'. Brenda listens, fascinated, to these people she barely knows. I end with the comment: 'This reveals at least as much about who they are, as who you are.'

Sometimes we get into situations in which our own transference reaction towards the other can be more intense and as a consequence it can hinder our actions. As if we have no other choice than to lapse into the behavioural pattern we recognise from the relationship with the person we associate with so strongly. In TA we speak of **rubber bands** that whisk us back to the past. All of a sudden it feels like we're standing in front of our father, mother, grandfather, grandmother or teacher, instead of, for instance, in front of the customs officer asking us to open our bag for a check at the airport. This example provides an insight into two important elements of psychological transference: situations in which an authority is concerned and/or tense situations. They are the triggers that easily get us to relapse into old behavioural patterns.

I bought a new suit last week. During the fitting I felt clumsy and shy, especially coming out of the fitting room to show my wife and the two shop assistants how it looked on me. It felt like I was walking into the living room at my parental home whilst my mother observed me critically and my brothers were joking and larking around.

In this situation my transference reaction hinders me so although I am 49, I am only able to behave like the six-year-old I used to be. At that moment, I put the faces of my mother and brothers, who used to play a role, on to the people in the present.

Assignment

Think of somebody you're in contact with who generates strong reactions in you: positive or negative.

Who does this person remind you of?

How are you triggered: something this person does, what they look like, smell like, feel like, the environment they are in or something else?
What do they do repeatedly? And then what do you do? How does it end?

The Pattern of Transference

Let us take a look back at the ego-states from Chapter 3. The ego states are very helpful in order to give us a better understanding of the pattern of transference. I'll briefly repeat what they are about so you don't have to look it up yourself.

As mentioned before, we have three ego-states at our disposal:

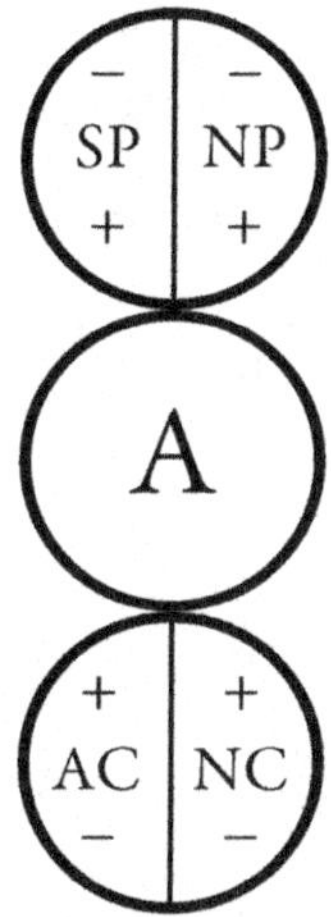

The Parent, in which we have stored behaviour, experiences, thoughts and feelings from parental figures. The Parent is divided into a Structuring Parent and a Nurturing Parent and both can be active in a positive or a negative way.

The Adult, in which behaviour, thoughts and feelings are based on the happenings in the here-and-now.

The Child, in which we have stored behaviour, thoughts and feelings from our childhood. The Child is divided into the Adapted Child and the Natural Child and both can be active in a positive or a negative way.

This can be illustrated as follows:

Both the Parent and the Child ego states are positions from which transference can take place. They are connected with both positive and negative experiences from the past.

As an example, let me return to Gerald and the problems he faces with his supervisor.

I ask Gerald what his supervisor does to make him react in such a strong way.
Gerald: He snaps at me whenever I haven't completed my work.

LK: And what happens to you when he does that?
Gerald: I feel he is treating me like a little boy, just like my father used to do.

LK: *And what happens next?*
Gerald: *Then I walk away in anger and I feel like slamming the door behind me.*
LK: *And what happens next?*
Gerald: *Well yeah, he gets even more disgruntled of course.*

Gerald's boss reacts to him in a way that Gerald's father possibly reacted when he didn't do what his father expected of him. Gerald's boss is also in transference.

Making use of the ego-states, the dialogue above can be illustrated as follows:

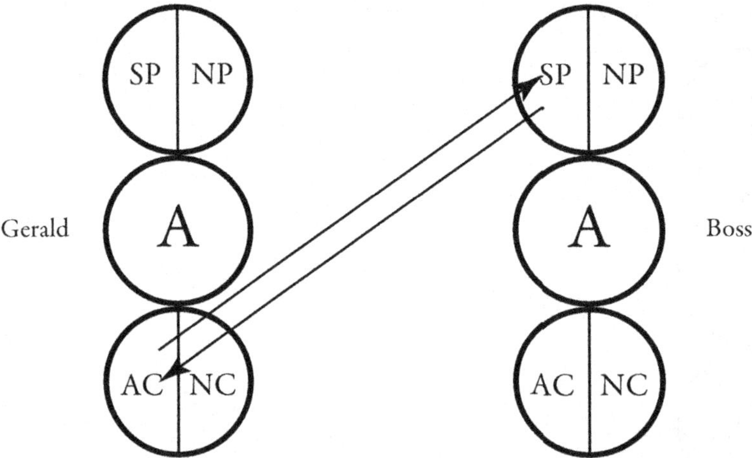

Gerald's boss is dissatisfied with Gerald's performance, which triggers him to react from the negative Structuring Parent. In turn Gerald counterreacts from the negative Adapted Child, and so on.

This pattern can perpetuate itself endlessly and consequently the individual perceptions of the worlds of both parties will continue to be reaffirmed. Gerald's perception of the world that 'bosses aren't to be trusted' will be reinforced and his boss' perception 'that employees need to be treated firmly' will also be reaffirmed. Although both beliefs have been developed in the past, they continue to be reinforced by current behaviour and the reaction that this provokes from others.

Assignment

Take another look at the transference relationship you thought of in the previous questions. Can you see the transaction pattern?

You can distinguish different kinds of transference. I will highlight two main categories.

Complementary transference – A projects the actual or historical parent onto B. Such is the case of Gerald when he 'puts the face' of his authoritarian father onto his boss.

Corresponding transference – A projects his or her own childhood feelings onto B allowing A to identify with B.

Geraldine feels sorry for her supervisor. She is getting a lot of criticism from her colleagues. Geraldine thinks that her supervisor must be feeling lonely. She recognises this feeling herself at times when she used to be rejected by her parents. She decides to buy her supervisor a nice piece of cake.

Transference is not always harmful. At times it can even temporarily be helpful to someone.

Steven liked to go to the professor's room at the faculty. The room is filled with books and he lov ed the smell of pipe tobacco. The professor projected the same kind of comfort and authority as his father. It felt just like it used to be at home.

However, over time, the positive transference relationship may get in the way of the development of your own autonomy.

Steven graduated years ago. He still ran all his publications by his former professor. It was as if he wanted his approval over and over again.

And transference can often be obstructive and sometimes even destructive.

Adrian recently started to tweet about his director's 'terrible behaviour'. He wished he could have had this kind of media back in the day to get even with his father.

Working on Your Own Transference Patterns

In Chapter 10 I talked about the importance of autonomy. Transference stands in the way of autonomy. It hinders you from choosing freely and acting in the here-and-now. After all, transference keeps on pulling you back to earlier life experiences and life positions. Transference is an invitation to repetition. That is why it is of interest to find out about your own transference patterns.

Assignment

> **Who or what arouses strong feelings inside you, positive or negative?**
> **Are these feelings commensurate with the situation? Or might they be too strong?**
> **If you are experiencing strong feelings: how can you connect the present (here-and-now) situation to past experiences?**

The situation as it presents itself isn't the same as the experience you had before. Put space between the here-and-now and the past. You can do this, for example, by:

> writing down your old experiences or sharing them with a good friend
> literally distancing yourself, viewing what is going on at a distance and figuring out how the situation differs from your earlier experience.
> using creative working methods: expressing the feeling in a painting or a poem.

If an experience keeps on recurring, it may help to seek out a coach or a counsellor. They can help you understand and change the complex processes of transference.

In the next chapter I will elaborate on these obstructive and destructive forms of transference relationships when I move on to the concept of games.

13. Games

That one may smile, and smile, and be a villain.

William Shakespeare, 'Hamlet', Act 1, Scene 5

The previous chapter was about transference. I described transference as a repetition of old relationship patterns in the present. In TA, every transference relationship is called a 'game', in the sense of psychological games. In Chapter 8, in which I talked about time structuring, I called this 'seeming intimacy'.

You can find numerous examples of games in plays or movies, such as the depressing play *Who's afraid of Virginia Woolf'* or more recently the movie *Carnage*. In both play and movie the characters seem to enter into some form of intimacy and then all of a sudden, unexpectedly, they lash out at each other.

This chapter gives you an overview of the different kinds of game and insight into the reason why people play games. This may help you explore the repetitive game patterns in your own life and also help you to change these patterns into healthier relationship patterns.

In contact people sometimes do things with an ulterior motive. The motive unexpectedly emerges when one of the parties show a sudden change of behaviour. Each person involved will then feel confused and misunderstood and will blame the other for this. The following example illustrates this process.

Chas walks up to his colleague Andrea and sits down with a sigh. Andrea pushes her chair back and asks Chas if there is anything she can do for him. The following dialogue then unfolds:

C: *I'm not getting anywhere with that client from Romford*
A: *How come?*
C: *(sigh) They keep on returning the documents to me with all kinds of comments.*
A: *You could give them a call.*
C: *(deeper sigh) Yes but they're always busy. I can never get them on the phone.*
A: *Perhaps it would be wise for you to drive down for a meeting.*
C: *Yes but that will take me all day.*
A: *Maybe it would be a good idea to talk it through with our team?*
C: *(a very deep sigh) Yes but then I'll get the speech that I'm not handling things well. (irritated) I can see that you're of no help.*

Chas trudges away leaving Andrea behind in amazement.

Let's take a closer look at this example making use of the ego states and the transactions for further analysis.

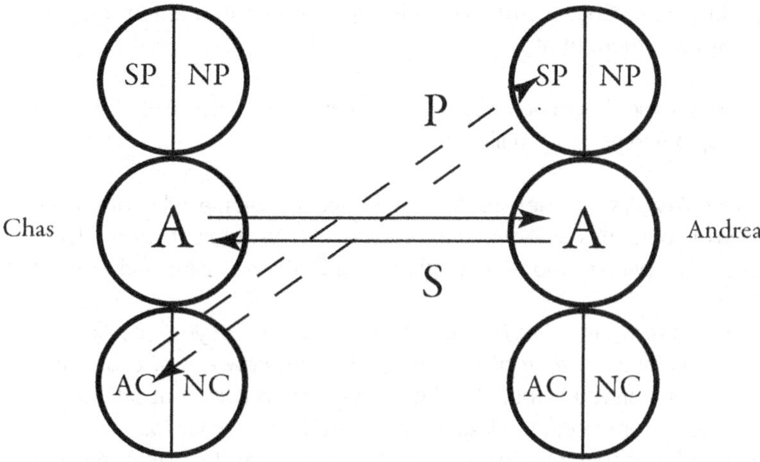

S = Social Level

P = Psychological Level

Chas asks for help from Adult at the social level. Or at least it looks like he's asking for help. Andrea replies from Adult at the social level. However, at the psychological level, a different kind of transaction is taking place. Chas takes on a helpless attitude (Child), whilst Andrea responds as if she knows what to do (Parent). Up till the point that the conversation changes when Chas gives Andrea the message that she is of no help.

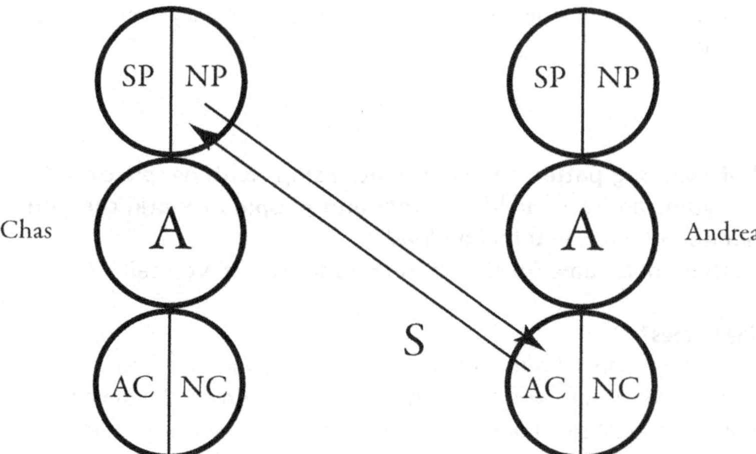

Suddenly Chas adds a new twist to the conversation and this is the point when his unconscious intention is revealed at the social level, namely giving Andrea the feeling that she is inadequate. In this example Chas is playing a classical TA game that is called 'Why Don't You, Yes But'. Andrea is also playing the game, because she is acting as if she can solve a problem that Chas is struggling with. She persists in offering solutions that Chas will already have thought of.

In TA a large number of games have been distinguished and all have been given colourful names. Let me sum up a few of them to illustrate:

> **Why does this Always Happen to Me?** – played by people who often feel Victimised, and of course by game 'partners' who seem to want to put people down.
> **Kick Me** – played by people who 'tempt' others to give them a 'slap', and by those who want to 'slap'.
> **Gotcha** *(you may see this in other TA books called Now I've Got you, you Son of a Bitch - that was not seen as a problem in the 1960s but now it is of course very politically incorrect)* – played by people who are seeking to catch out others, and by 'partners' who are pretending to know more than they really know.
> **Harried** – played by people who want others to believe that they are dominated by work and that they are unable to do anything about it, and by others who continue to give them so much work without ever querying.
> **Ain't It Awful** – played by people who like to gossip, and then one or other of them may suddenly criticise the 'partner' for being so negative.
> **I'm Only Trying to Help You** – played by people who offer help that is not needed and then get upset when the help is rejected.
> **Millstone** – played by people who make excuses about their inadequacies when there is no real reason why they could not do something.

In this kind of social process between people, over and over again, the initial message at the social level is not in line with the message at the psychological level and all of a sudden the tone of the interaction will change. In addition, I should like to emphasise that people play games out of awareness. At the moment it is happening they actually feel that their own feelings are authentic.

Assignment

> **What kind of recurring patterns in your relationships with people close to you, such as your family, your life partner and people at work, can you identify, that end up with you feeling 'bad'?**
> **If you could think of a name for this pattern, what would you call it?**

Why Do People Play Games?

Games involve the reinforcement of your script and your life position. You repeat an old pattern and think: *Ah, there you are, you see, it just shows you....* And at the same time, by doing that you avoid difficult situations in which there is a real need for contact. The game may seem to be intimate such as in the case of Andrea who feels that she can help Chas. In addition, the game provides for many (negative) strokes and that is sometimes preferable to getting none at all. Finally, it gives people a lot to talk about. A lot goes on. That's why many people love to watch soap operas as a popular pastime because these are all made up of game situations.

There are of course some games which are played very commonly and the consequences do not seem to be too bad. However, life is better if we learn how to avoid playing games because that means we are having more straightforward relationships with people.

Assignment

Take a look at your own example above and think about how you are tempted to step into this pattern over and over again.
And how come the same thing happens to the other person(s)?

When a game is going on, an old pattern is being repeated. The players are moving on familiar terrain and act in a way that they have learned and are familiar with from childhood. They are thus continuing to recreate transference situations. And by doing so, they reinforce their life position (+-/-+/--).

During her childhood Carol felt that there was hardly any space for herself. At school she increasingly exhibited problem behaviour, which led to her being expelled from school three times in a row. Soon after she started her first job she got into a quarrel with her employer. She felt she was being treated unfairly. She got fired and got three new jobs after that, but every time she was sent away within the trial period.

Degrees of Games

Three levels of games can be distinguished:

First degree games – will cause social embarrassment. These kinds of games are quite common. They occur in many relationships, at home, at work and with friends.

She: Tidy up your own clothes for a change!
He: It's not like I don't want to tidy them up, you just never give me a chance to do it myself!
She: Yeah right, now it's my fault!

Second degree games – the game has a major social consequence such as the loss of one's job or the termination of a relationship.

After cheating on her husband for the third time, she messed up her second marriage too.

Third degree games – the game causes massive damage and can end up either in major violence, in the courtroom or in prison.

Every evening after returning home from the pub he would beat up his son. In the morning he would express his deepest regrets in tears.

Over time games tend to increase in severity. A humble beginning can steadily escalate. It goes from bad to worse. And when looking back in time, often something innocuous will seem to have been the cause of it.

The two colleagues were making each other's lives miserable. They kept on sending each other nasty e-mails and cc-ing the entire team. And during meetings they kept on slinging the same retorts back and forth. When one day they were yelling at each other in the street in front of their office, it was obviously the last straw for their other colleagues. In the conversations that followed it became clear that one of them didn't feel that he was being taken seriously whilst the other felt scared by the excessive reaction that this apparently caused. It had evolved into a profound distrust. A distrust that continued to grow....

The Drama Triangle

Games are created by repetitive patterns. Stephen Karpman developed the so-called Drama Triangle as another way of making these patterns visible. This is a widely known TA concept, frequently used by people who do not know anything about TA.

The Drama Triangle can be used as an instrument in order to map out ineffective patterns and barriers to communication. Using the Drama Triangle you can explore frustrating situations in which you are going round in circles without getting anywhere. What's going wrong and what is the cause of it? What am I doing and why am I doing it? What is the other person doing and what effect does that have on me?

And then, most importantly: what can I do to get out of it?

The Drama Triangle can be seen as a source of support for you to choose how you would like to respond.

The Drama Triangle has three roles: the Persecutor, the Rescuer and the Victim. In the following example I have placed the various roles between the brackets.

Charles talks to his supervisor about the problems he's having with his colleague Pauline. Charles is upset (Victim) because Pauline has offended him (Persecutor) for not getting the job done. Charles explains emotionally that things are extremely chaotic at home as he is moving and that he is therefore having difficulty in managing things at work (Victim). Peter (Rescuer). promises to discuss this with Pauline. During the break he handles the matter sensitively, but Pauline (Persecutor). gets furious and accuses him of making excuses for Charles. She is angry because 'Charles isn't committed to the cause and Peter always covers for him'. Peter loses control and walks away. He feels he has failed both his employees for not solving the problem. At home he complains about how tough his job is (Victim).

In the situation described above you can distinguish the following three roles: the Rescuer, the Victim and the Persecutor. The three roles point to ineffective behaviour that in turn maintains the negative situation. In the Drama Triangle a role change occurs at a switch. In this example, for instance, Peter switches from Rescuer to Victim.

A small boy who falls into the water not being able to swim is a real victim and needs a rescuer; somebody to help him get out of the water safely. If someone were to jump into the water and cry out for help even though they can swim, we would think of them as a Victim for not using their own abilities. Obviously, pretending not to be able to swim would be a strange thing to do. But people frequently act as if they cannot do things when they can, and other people then reinforce that by trying to help them instead of prompting them to work out their own solutions.

Assignment

Which abilities are Charles, Peter and Pauline neglecting to use?

The Drama Triangle can be used to analyse situations in which games occur. What are the various roles being played by the participants in the game? Games can be played both in pairs, in threes and in groups.

Jasper had been kicked out of the group of boys. They were always picking on him. The girls felt sorry for Jasper and they were therefore very sweet to him. Until the day he threw one of the girl's schoolbags into the rubbish bin. Although this deed gained him the regard of some of the boys, he lost the goodwill of the girls. From that time on the girls bullied him relentlessly.

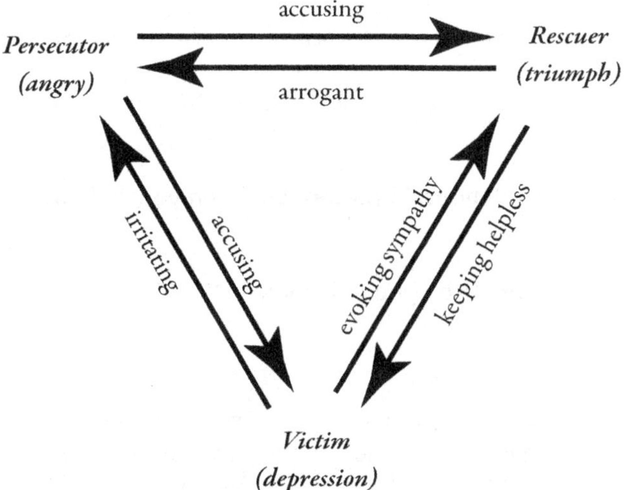

Drama Triangle

The Rescuer loves to help others. They get fulfilment from caring for others. They think, act and feels for others without checking, keeping the others dependent.. The Rescuer doesn't bear in mind that it is necessary to have a fair balance in a relationship. The Rescuer works hard, but eventually their help will prove ineffective and often it will be resented.

Maureen is always the first person to give advice, even before you've asked for any.

Jeff asked his neighbour if he would empty his letterbox whilst he was away on holiday. When Jeff returns he notices to his annoyance that his neighbour had not only emptied the letterbox, but had also put up new hooks next to his coat rack. His neighbour explains: 'I'm so sorry, but I was in your house and I wasn't making any use of the hooks anyway.'

The Victim has a problem, feels helpless and discounts their own power and qualities. They call upon the help of others and assume that other people will solve their problem.

Frank is falling behind with his work. He tells his supervisor that he can't do anything about it. 'My supplies aren't being delivered on time and furthermore it's a lot of work for one person and nobody wants to help me.'

Maragret's bicycle has been standing in the shed for weeks with a flat tire. She complains to her mother that she doesn't know what to do. 'I can't fix the tire and I can't walk all the way to the bicycle repairman, can I?'

The Persecutor has an embittered, accusing and vindictive attitude. They blame others for events that occur, which gives them some relief but only in the short-term.

Karin runs her fingers along the skirting board and then points her finger accusingly in the direction of the cleaning lady, who has been busy with other tasks: 'Not properly cleaned again!'

Bert refuses to pay alimony after the divorce. 'She brought it on herself, the bitch', he can't resist telling his friends. 'That'll teach her.'

Assignment

Take another look at an undesirable relationship pattern between yourself and another person.

> **Which position in the Drama Triangle do you initially take?**
> **And what do they take?**
> **How does it evolve?**

One of the features of the Drama Triangle is that you are, as it were, held in prison, albeit the prison that you yourself have created. The various roles create suction. They complement each other and neither one can do without the other. One person's 'choice' of role will determine the other person's 'choice' of role. If one is the Rescuer, then the others will become Persecutors or Victims. The roles may also collide, for instance when two Persecutors berate each other or when two Rescuers give each other consolation. Every conceivable combination of roles can occur. As the interaction unfolds, it won't take long before the participants switch roles.

There was a big conflict going on between the board members. During meetings they badmouthed each other. One board member portrayed the other as 'unreliable', whilst the other board member accused her colleague of being 'a money-grabber'. Both of them complained to their colleagues about how much they were suffering from the distorting behaviour of their colleague. 'It's impossible for me to sleep at night because of the hurtful way he/she is behaving towards me.'

The Drama Triangle is a dynamic model: people rarely stay in one role. You move around the triangle from one role to the other. A Victim will seek out a Rescuer, but after a while will take on the role of the Persecutor if it turns out that the Rescuer is not able to solve the problems. The Rescuer will then become the Victim ('Nothing I do is good enough, I'm a useless counsellor'), but after a while the Victim becomes Persecutor in order to take revenge and accuse the other ('It's all your own fault').

We often change roles in different contexts. At work we may be our clients' Rescuers. We may be Persecutors towards all colleagues who aren't committed to the client or to the CEO who doesn't reward our efforts. Subsequently we go home exhausted and start complaining like the Victim about how work is draining energy out of us and that we don't know what to do about it. However, it should be noted that everyone has a favourite position in the Drama Triangle, which is usually based on your own history. It is the role that you 'easily' slide into at times you feel under pressure.

Assignment

Which role in the Drama Triangle do you know best?

The Bystanders
Over time, a valuable addition has been made to the original concept: the role of the Bystander(s). There's no drama without Bystanders.

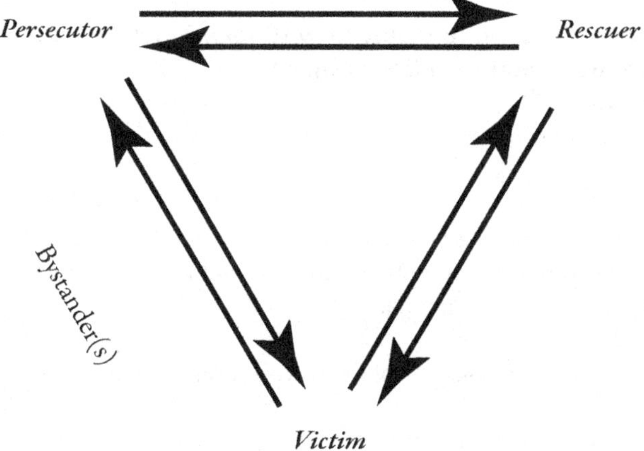

Drama Triangle and bystander(s)

That is to say that many 'players' in the drama Triangle take on their role specifically because of the presence of bystanders. You can imagine the employee walking up to his boss to complain about a colleague just as he sees that his other colleagues could hear what he had to say. He consciously speaks louder for dramatic effect.

In a meeting, two people start an argument which becomes more and more heated, and what is being said moves into personal insults rather than logical comments. Everyone else at the meeting watches. Some of them are feeling frustrated at the waste of time, some of them feel a bit scared as the comments escalate, and some of them think it makes the meeting more exciting to have this to watch. No-one intervenes to stop the argument.

The Bystander is a passive role. As a spectator they watch and at most, often subconsciously, their facial expressions will show approval or disapproval. The presence of Bystanders intensifies the game.

As usual, Bernard is pushing Gerald around. Bernard is mocking and making fun of him. During break he puts salt in his coffee and makes a mess of his desk. The other colleagues stand by and watch.

The colleagues in this example are part of the game. Their passivity contributes to the continuation and the enhancement of the game. They can either choose to continue to play a passive role and stay part of the problem, or start to contribute towards a solution.

One day, Karen walks up to Bernard. 'I would like to ask you to stop being nasty to Gerald. If you have a problem with him, then you should discuss it directly with him. This is harassment and it's about time that it stops. It's causing a bad atmosphere in our department.' This helped to break the negative pattern.

Assignment

> **Have you recently been in a situation (possibly unwittingly) in which you took on the Bystander's role in other people's 'drama'?**
> **How could you have intervened?**
> **What prevented you from intervening?**

The Winner's Triangle

No doubt each and every one of us regularly gets 'sucked' into a game, not to say daily. It is difficult to avoid, considering the complexity of human communication. It is therefore above all a matter of finding ways to step out of the game.

In order to develop options for this you could make use of the so-called Winner's Triangle.

In the Winner's Triangle you make use of the life position 'I'm OK, you're OK.' Therefore, the first question you are facing is: 'How to get back to this life position?' In Chapter 11 I already gave you some suggestions. I will summarise these briefly again.

You yourself are +

> **Give yourself the message that you are OK just the way you are.**
> **Ask for positive strokes and give yourself strokes.**
> **Be active and focus on your life goals.**
> **Pay attention to your stance: remember to always ground yourself and be in contact with the world around you.**

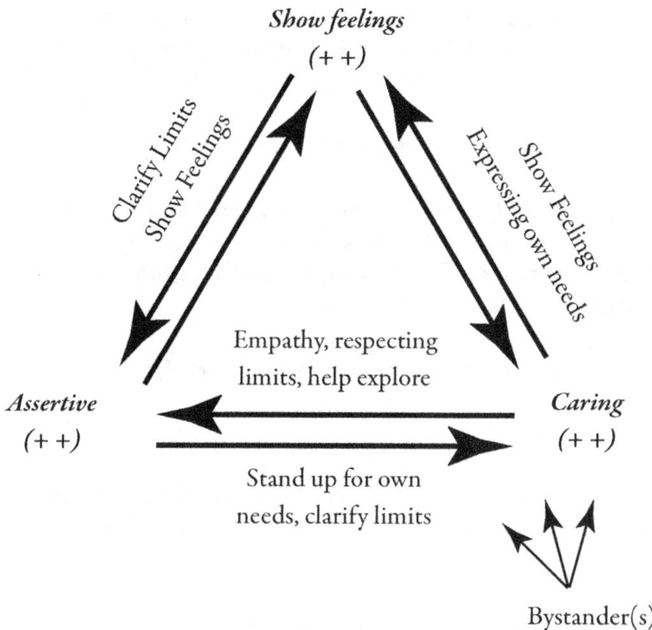

The Winner's Triangle

The other is +

Practice expressing your appreciation for others.
Let go of a too strong focus on performance.
Have fun with yourself and others.
Practice looking kind and gentle in front of the mirror.

Maintaining + +

Take good care of yourself and others.
Ask yourself whether you and others are benefitting from your actions.
Be assertive. Stand up for your own interests and those of others.
Pay attention to both task and relationship.
Enjoy.

In addition, you have an arsenal of behaviour at your disposal that can help you step out of the Drama Triangle:

Show your feelings - it is in the interest of yourself and others to show your own authentic feelings (Afraid, Angry, Happy, Sad) and express your needs.

Be assertive - furthermore, it is important that both you and others are clear on your own boundaries and stand up for your own needs.

Caring - finally, it is in your own interest and the interest of the other person that you take care of them, that you respect their boundaries and help them explore situations for their own benefit.

I have combined this behavioural repertoire into one example:

For weeks now Mark has been quarrelling with Lucia. He feels hurt and belittled because she had been having an affair with another man behind his back. In the meantime, Lucia feels really guilty. Every now and then she lashes out to him. That evening, whilst fighting for the umpteenth time, Lucia looks at Mark:

Lucia: *I would like to end this trench war we're in. It's making me sad and I feel hurt.*

Mark: *What about me?*

Lucia: *Yes, I can see you're hurt and sad and I understand. And I want to offer you my sincerest regret. I just want us to talk about it and stop making each other's lives miserable.*

Mark: *(who is finding it hard to let go of the game): Look before you leap . . .*

Lucia: *Mark, stop it!*

Mark: *(silence)*

Lucia: *I get that I have hurt you. And I am extremely sorry. I have crossed the line and I shouldn't have. I would really like to talk to you to see if there is anything I can do to heal the damage. And I would also like to explore together with you how this could have happened in our relationship. Would you like to do that?*

Mark: *(cries)*

Lucia: *(takes his hand)*

Lucia and Mark have taken a first great step. After all, the journey begins with the willingness of both parties to step out of the Drama Triangle.

Assignment

> **Are there times when you hold on to your hurt feelings?**
> **What are you gaining for keeping it like this?**
> **What costs do you pay for keeping it like this?**
> **Is it worth the costs?**

It's often hard to free yourself from a destructive pattern. Because you are hurt, you easily experience that you are the one who is right. And that makes it hard to step out of the Drama Triangle. We then often need help from outsiders (Bystanders). They can set things in motion by stepping out of the 'spectator seat' and actually starting to contribute actively towards the solution.

Carol, Lucia's best friend, had a firm talk with Lucia that afternoon: 'You'll have to face Mark at some time instead of hiding and wallowing in self-loathing. That won't solv e anything, neither for you, or Mark or your relationship.' This helped Lucia cross the threshold.

It's hard to step out of the Drama Triangle by yourself.

14. Symbiosis

It is the curse of kings to be attended by slaves.

William Shakespeare, 'King John', Act 4, Scene 2

In this chapter I will elaborate on an important mechanism that is part of games: symbiosis. Within symbiotic relationships people have difficulty standing on their own two feet. They become dependent on each other. In the development of your own autonomy it is important that you learn to recognise symbiotic relationships, to discover why you enter into relationships in this way and to learn to relate in a different and beneficial way. This is what this chapter is about.

Unhealthy symbiosis is a breeding ground for games.

Symbiosis
The term symbiosis is firmly established in biology and medicine. In Greek sym means "together" and bios means "life" as in living together. Good examples of this can be found in nature.

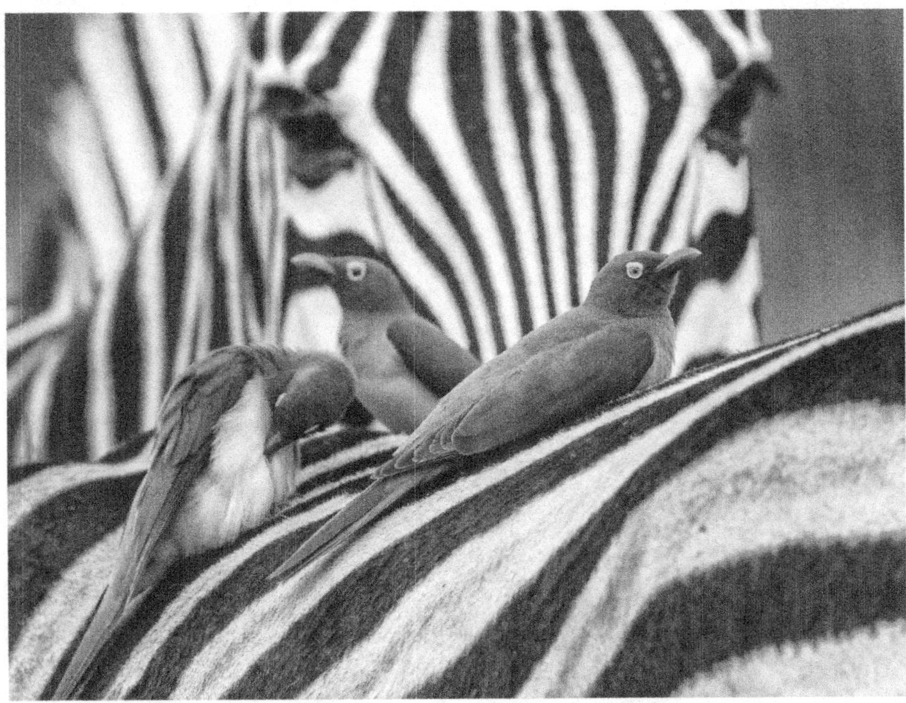

The birds pick off the parasites from the back of the zebra. The zebra gets rid of the parasites and the birds satisfy their hunger.

The term symbiosis is also used within psychology. Symbiosis occurs when two or more individuals behave as though they constitute a single person.

Astrid's daughter Vera is two years old. Vera can walk on her own, but she is not yet able to handle traffic. She can feed herself, but she is not yet able to cook and do the dishes. She can sit up in the bath without help, but is not yet able to make sure the water is at the right temperature. Astrid takes care of all the things that Vera is not yet able to do.

We all have experienced symbiosis in this way during our upbringing, when it was healthy because the needs were genuine. However, symbiotic traits tend to re-occur within many later relationships in the sense that partners tend to take over certain functions in life.

She takes care of the financial papers for both of them, whilst he plans out the holidays.

The symbiosis becomes unhealthy when it undermines the autonomy of those involved. The choice to behave becomes limited considering the fact that the partners keep on repeating patterns. This is a breeding ground for games.

Edward has always been 'the strong man' in their relationship who has a solution for everything. His wife Jean has always been 'the vulnerable woman' who needs the strong man to lean upon and keep on going.

Assignment

Can you give an example of a healthy symbiosis from your own life?
And can you give an example of an unhealthy symbiosis?

When symbiosis occurs within a relationship, the people involved discount certain parts of themselves. In the example above, Edward is discounting the vulnerable part of himself, whilst Jean is discounting her ability to stand on her own two feet. A key element in this is that the Adult awareness about what is adequate in the here-and-now is (partly) missing.

At a deeper psychological level a reverse pattern is taking place.

This subject arose during a conv ersation with Jean and Edward. I ask Jean what would happen if she were to stand on her own two feet. Her answer is short and unequivocal: 'Oh well, Edward wouldn't be able to handle that. He needs to take care of me.'

At a subconscious, psychological level, Jean is taking care of Edward by remaining dependent on him in order for Edward to keep on feeling big and strong.

People get into these kinds of symbiotic relationships because they haven't (yet) been able to resolve certain issues from the past with their own parents or other relationships. As a consequence the symbiotic relationship gets acted out once more. This provides a sense of security and it also reinforces the life script. In this context you might want to think back about the stages of development described in Chapter 1 and how certain developmental tasks are related to the various stages of development. If a certain developmental task has not been completed, you will be faced with it later in your life. In this respect, transference always plays an important role within symbiotic relationships.

As a child, Jean didn't get a chance to stand on her own two feet. Her mother kept her on a tight leash. Her mother made all the decisions for her, whether in relation to the kind of clothes she should wear or the school she should go to. In her relationship with Edward she came up against the same problem, which led her to make herself dependent on him.

Assignment

> **Which repetitive relationship pattern do you recognise in the example of the unhealthy symbiosis you thought of earlier?**
> **Which developmental task lies before you?**

Passive Behaviour

A symbiotic relationship can be recognised by four types of passive behaviour, one or more of which will apply.. The behaviour is called passive because it does not give rise to solving the problem or issue. You display this kind of behaviour when you are not willing to take responsibility and you want to stay in a dependent relationship.

1. **Doing nothing** occurs when someone does not act or does not respond.
   Gerald is late for an appointment. Martin confronts him with this and tells him that he is annoyed. Gerald just looks at him without saying a word.

2. **Over-adaption** occurs when people 'blindly' comply with the goals, desires and expectations of others. Or they already imagine what the other person wants after which they adjust their behaviour accordingly. Over-adaption is a behaviour that is often seen as a nice and generous quality in a person, who will often be appreciated for it.
   Patricia feels like going into town to find a nice sunny sidewalk café to sit at. As soon as Peter asks her to mend his trousers, she, as usual, lets go of her own plan and gets to work.

3. **Agitation** can be recognised by repetitive, purposeless behaviour. Agitated people experience unpleasant inner turmoil and try to discharge the inner tension by making agitated moves, of which they are usually not aware.
   The director looked friendly, but her employees could tell by the way she was kicking her leg under the table that things were taking too long and she was getting annoyed.

4. **Incapacitation (inward) or violence (outward)**: two forms in which the energy that has been built up in the previous three phases gets discharged. When this happens, others around seem to accept that the individual cannot be expected to deal with life and have to do it for them.
   After a long day of meetings Astrid always wound up with a migraine. This meant her colleagues had to do some of her work.

From one moment to the other Bryan could start shouting and screaming. He would fling everything around he could get hold of. This meant that his colleagues backed off and left him alone.

Assignment

Think of an example in which you displayed passive behaviour.

>**What type of behaviour did you display?**
>**What did you do?**
>**What did you get out of it?**

Discounting

In an unhealthy symbiosis discounting is always involved. When a person is discounting, they unawarely ignore some aspect of:

Self
When Patricia immediately started to mend Peter's trousers, she discounted her own desire to sit at a sunny sidewalk café.

Others
When Gerald was late for his appointment and didn't respond to Martin's being annoyed, he discounted Martin's justified irritation.

The situation
When the director was kicking her leg agitatedly, she was discounting the need to talk things through before making a decision.

Assignment

Think back on the unhealthy symbiotic relationship pattern you conjured up earlier.

>**Are you discounting yourself?**
>**Others?**
>**The situation?**

Discounting can occur at various levels:

The existence of a situation or problem
Patricia wasn't even aware that as soon as Peter opened his mouth, she would go running.

The significance of the situation or problem
When she spoke to her friends about her relationship with Peter, they were surprised to hear about Patricia's lack of own space. Patricia wasn't able to relate to that: 'It doesn't matter'.

The changeability of the situation or problem
After a few months Patricia started to feel uncomfortable. She talked it over with her mother and her conviction stayed the same: 'That's just how it goes in relationships between men and women. And there's no changing that.'

One's own ability to change
One day Patricia's best friend told her about the positive changes in her relationship, in which her boyfriend had taken on a much larger part of the household chores. Patricia just sighed and said that she was glad for her friend, but that she herself could never be capable of doing that. She simply wouldn't be able to stand up to Peter.

Discounting always takes place out of awareness. The Adult ego-state is simply not joining the party.

Exaggeration
Discounting always goes hand in hand with exaggeration. An aspect is being discounted partly because another aspect is getting an exaggerated amount of attention.

Patricia told her friend about Peter's extreme clumsiness. 'He's like a baby, but a 6 ft tall one.'

Because Patricia wants to emphasise Peter's clumsiness in this example, she exaggerates: Peter is not a baby anymore, but a grown man. By exaggerating she is discounting the fact that Peter is an adult.

Working with Discounting and Exaggeration
To help you get started to work on your own discounting and exaggerations, either by yourself or with the help of someone else, you can make use of a simple road map, which I will explain on the basis of Peter and Patricia's example.

Step 1: Recognition of the facts: what's going on?
Patricia is talking to her best friend about her relationship with Peter. In the course of the conversation Patricia starts to pick up on a number of things. She acknowledges that she manages the household and is almost always the one doing the chores.

Step 2: Recognition of the significance: How come this is a problem?
Patricia then acknowledges that she is making Peter more and more dependent on her and that she herself is getting out of the house less and less and that she hardly sees her friends any more.

Step 3: Recognition of the desirability to do something about the problem: how necessary is it to solve the problem?
Patricia feels that by continuing to behave in the same way, she is increasingly isolating herself. In addition, her relationship with Peter is getting tense. She realises that she needs to do something about it or otherwise her relationship might end up on the rocks.

Step 4: Recognition of the possibility to do something about it: am I capable of doing anything?
She realises that she first needs to talk things over with Peter and that she can also arrange to meet up with her friends and spend some time with them.

Step 5: Recognition of the capacity to create successful change: do I have the knowledge and the skills to change things? Or do I need to seek for them elsewhere?
Patricia is dreading the awkward talk with Peter. At the same time she knows that she is strong enough to deal with it. They have always been able to have good conversations in the past. And she also has the skills to talk to people about difficult issues, that she has learned to do in her job as a social worker.

Step 6: Recognition of the commitment to change: am I going for it?
She decides to go for it and she feels strong enough. Her best friend tells her that she has never seen such determination in her before and she wishes her good luck and success.

Use the steps above to explore your own unhealthy symbiosis example.

Intermezzo

During a following group session we explore Christine's behavioural pattern: the quiet, closed supervisor from the building company, who in an earlier session had shared some of her childhood experiences (see the Prologue). We investigate the pattern on the basis of the position she has taken within the supervision group.

On her own initiative, Christine starts talking about why she always keeps at a distance from others: 'I never feel I have anything of significance to contribute. I don't feel I have anything worthwhile to say, only if it's about my work. I derive my sense of security from my professional knowledge. At least that is one area in which I feel safe. When it comes to human relationships, like now, I feel clumsy and stupid and I'm afraid of being exposed.'

I ask the other group members what effect Christine's closed posture has on them:

B: *I always feel a bit scared of you. I haven't a clue what is going on in your head and that makes me feel insecure.*
D: *I always feel I want to help you and that you're not able to make it on your own. Like the last time during our conversation I find myself almost wanting to tell you what to say and I feel very sorry for you.*
K: *I really feel the urge to give you a good shake when you keep your mouth shut and act clumsily. I would rather turn around and walk away.*

Christine listens to what is being said with increasing amazement. 'I can't believe I evoke all these things in you!' We then talk about transference and I ask B, D and K to each explore their own transference in relation to Christine: how come Christine's attitude brings about such strong emotions within you?

After some explanation and some additional questions, all three of them are able to give an answer:

B: *You're just like my grandmother. A quiet person who was always angry and who I was afraid of.*

D: *You remind me of myself, how I used to be. Quiet, shy, insecure. I wish somebody would have helped me back then.*

K: *I hate people with closed postures. Since I was a child I was told that you should stand firmly on your own feet. There was no room for that wait-and-see attitude like yours. You would have gotten a kick in the pants a number of times for doing that.*

We then further explore these reactions with use of the Drama Triangle. B, D and K each recognise the position they have taken.

B: Victim
D: Rescuer
K: Persecutor

Christine recognises herself as the Victim. She slowly begins to understand that from B's perspective (the only man in the group), she could also be in the position of the Persecutor. Then suddenly she starts to chuckle: 'At last I understand why they offered me a management position at the building company, if that is the impact I have on men!'

During the next session they figure out which life position each of them have adopted on the basis of the 'window on the world'. Again we use Christine's situation as 'practice material'. Christine positions herself in the 'I'm not OK, you're OK' quadrant. 'But' she adds: 'At work I compensate for that. At work I'm OK and the others are not!' Together we explore Christine's options in order for her to shift to the OK-OK quadrant.

Christine tells us that this exercise is of extreme help to her.

LK: *How is it helping you?*
C: *In a kind and helpful way you have all invited me to share my story.*
LK: *What impact does that have?*
C: *It makes me feel calm.*
LK: *How does this happen within you?*
C: *I look at myself at a distance. I am able to get an overview of the situation and that makes me less afraid. And I can also come up with the idea that I am doing pretty well.*
B: *(adds) After all, you've been through such a great deal in your life and to me this is worth sharing.*
C: *Thank you.*

Christine has now found a place within the group in which she can safely experiment with new behaviour. She can show both her vulnerability and her strength. She can experience being nurtured by her colleagues. She is making use of the opportunity to expand to a wider range of behavioural patterns, which will help her become more effective at work.

For the development of your own autonomy it is important that you learn to recognise symbiotic relationships, to understand why you enter into such relationships and learn how to do things differently.

Epilogue:
About the free choice for development

15. Vital energy and courage to live

That which hath made them drunk made me bold, what hath

quench'd them hath given me fire.

William Shakespeare, 'Macbeth', Act 2, Scene 2

Stephanie was sacked and had a burn out. She stayed at home all day and barely let anybody in. She weighed 20 stone. One evening she was watching a program on T.V. that showed how people were getting their lives back into the saddle. She decides to get in touch with a nutritionist and an employment agency. Now, after six months, she's sitting in front of me. Beaming with pleasure she shows me a photo of herself from the time she was overweight. Within half a year she was able to lose 6 stone. She has recently started her own business and she hands over her business card to me. Enthusiastically she tells me about the successful business deal she had made that morning.

For a long time now Eric has been yearning to sing music from Bach. His busy job is preventing him from doing it. Up till the day that he simply decides not to procrastinate any longer and to sign up for singing lessons and join a choir.

These two examples are part of a long list of all kinds of examples that I have experienced in the last 25 years. Examples of people who have dared to connect their vital energy (Physis) to their courage to live (Thymos). This is closely linked with the last question of the previous chapter: are you going for it?

The story about Physis as shared with you in Chapter 1, is brimming over with optimism; an optimism that doesn't always get acknowledged. Looking at the world around me, I often see people dissatisfied with what they are doing, not having the courage to break away from things they are familiar with.

Courage always goes hand in hand with fear. Fear of not belonging, fear of not being able to manage in life, fear of guilt, fear of...?

Assignment

Are there things that are preventing you from doing what you really would like to do?

The root cause for you not doing the things you would like to do lies in your script, which is apparently restricting your growth. It takes a challenging quest to find the way out. In this book I have mainly focused on how people get caught up in their own personal history and how to break these patterns. It's all about uncovering the possibilities within yourself in order to part with patterns that aren't serving you. The word un-cover is a great word within the entire context. You already have the answer, you only have to take the cover off.

Sometimes we uncover great things, but usually it's about smaller things, like Eric and his desire to sing in a choir.

Without fear it is not possible to change. Change largely has to do with having the courage to face the fear. Fear of the unknown can become anxiety. Anxiety is about specific things with no specific threat. You are able to anticipate specific things, giving you the possibility to come up with a way to deal with the anxiety. What you are anxious about often appears to be smaller than what you were afraid of in the first place.

Monique had been working as a secretary for 15 years. She frequently felt depressed and lonely. Our conversations were often about her desire to let go of everything and make a new start. I invited her to make her fantasies more tangible and to explore whether they could lead to real options. At that time she was often afraid of the consequences. But her fear decreased as time went by and her plans became more specific. Recently I received a photo she had sent me from the Canary Islands, where she had moved three years ago, now working as a tour guide. On the back of the photo she had written how she loves every minute of it, that she was doing extremely well and that she was glad that she had found the courage to make the choice she had made.

Assignment

> **What do you dream of?**
> **Can you specify your dream?**
> **What does that look like?**
> **What is preventing you from achieving your dream?**

And that is how all of us eventually have the power to take off our masks, take off our make-up and get up on the stage, stand in the spotlights and say: **'THIS IS ME!'**

> *And the clock says tick, tick, tick*
> *Ticks changeless hours away*
> *For who always waits*
> *Comes everything always too late*

Translation of the song by Thé Lau, The Scene, 'Rigoureus'

tick, tick, tick, tick

For those of you who are curious to learn more

Sources of inspiration

The Prologue

Carl Jung has written many inspiring books on the (collective) unconscious. I derive my thoughts around 'the perfect and the full life' from his impressive study *Answer to Job*, a study on the roots of Christianity.

Friedrich Nietzsche's commonly used phrase 'become who you are' originates from his book *The Gay Science.*

In his book *Ben ik in beeld (Am I in the picture)*, Roek Lips writes about the social media in this day and age, pleading for openness in the media sector. During a number of personal conversations, we spoke at some length about the flip side of this openness, which gave me input for this prologue.

Chapter 1 - Vital Energy

In addition to Berne, Petruska Clarkson has written about 'Physis', for instance, in her book *Transactional Analysis Psychotherapy; an Integrated Approach*, which is, although not simple, very much worth reading.

Muriel James, an early student of Eric Berne, published a number of books in which she made the connection between TA and spirituality, such as in *Passion for Life.*

The 'aquarium' exercise was inspired by Giles Barrow's work. Giles is an educationalist and Transactional Analyst in the UK. You can download a variety of his articles from his website: www.educational-ta.net

Transactional Analysis isn't the only psychoanalytical theory that is based on the belief that people are able to grow and develop. TA belongs to the humanistic psychology school of thought that also considers the human ability to grow as an important starting point. In case you are interested in this way of thinking, it could be worthwhile for you to read Victor Frankl's work in particular. Frankl, a Jewish psychiatrist who had survived the Holocaust during the Second World War, was the developer of Logotherapy: a method founded upon the belief that it is the striving to find a meaning in one's life that is the primary, most powerful motivating and driving force in human beings The most accessible piece of work is his introductory book *Man's search for meaning*.

Chapter 2 - Bonding and Development

Within the fields of psychology and pedagogy, a lot of research has been done on bonding. John Bowlby is the most well-known and talked-about researcher on the subject. He wrote the three-part series *Attachment, Separation and Loss*.

The American writer Judith Viorst wrote an accessible book titled *Necessary Losses: The Loves Illusions Dependencies and Impossible Expectations That All of us Have*. She describes our path of life to be one of continuous farewells.

George Kohlrieser has authored quite a number of books on bonding. In his wonderful book *Hostage at the Table* he reveals how he applied the bonding principles in hostage negotiation and he uses this bonding process as a metaphor in normal everyday life. I have taken the bonding cycle from his work.

Riet Fiddelaars-Jaspers also used the bonding cycle as a basis for her beautiful book *Met mijn ziel onder de arm*.

The parts in which I have written about development are based on Pamela Levin's work. In her book *Cycles of Power* she describes the cycles of development. She has been inspired by Freud, Erikson and in particular Piaget's work. Unlike Piaget, she extends a person's development past the stage of adolescence and she describes the continuing cyclical nature of development. For years she carried out research into this development within her own, American, culture as well as within other cultures. The principles and staging proved to be universal. In order to clarify this universality, she used a quotation from the *I Ching*, part of which I have copied below:

'The idea of return is based on the course of nature. The movement is cyclic, and the course completes itself. Therefore it is not necessary to hasten anything artificially. Everything comes of itself at the appointed time. This is the meaning of heaven and earth. All movements are accomplished in six stages, and the seventh brings return.'

Chapters 3 and 4 - Ego-States and In Conversation with Ego-States

Eric Berne once said that you should be able to explain all aspects of TA on the basis of ego-states. Therefore, there is hardly a book about TA that does not mention at least something about ego-states.

Eric Berne himself wrote a lot about ego-states. He started out by writing a series of articles on intuition at the beginning of the 1950's. These articles were later brought together in a book titled *Intuition and Ego States*. Subsequently he wrote more on this subject in his books *What Do You Say After You Say Hello?* and *Games People Play*.

In 1993 the *Transactional Analysis Journal* (TAJ) published Pearl Drego's research article in which she describes a large variety of types of the ego state model; 27 (!) different interpretations of the model to be precise. No doubt some more have been added in the meantime, perhaps driving an outsider to despair. Apparently, the model can be explained and applied in so many different ways. For those who are interested in this subject I can recommend the book *Ego States* edited by Charlotte Sills and Helena Hargaden: heavy-going material for connoisseurs.

Chapter 5 - A Closer look at The Adult Ego-State

My own thinking on ego states is mainly based on Keith Tudor's writings on the integrating Adult in the book *Ego States (Key Concepts in Transactional Analysis)*. In addition, Susannah Temple's work is an exceptional source of inspiration for me. Her articles can be downloaded via the website www.functionalfluency.com.

I derived the learning curve from work done by Piet Weisfelt and Wibe Veenbaas. However, the origin of the model is lost in the mists of time – it may even go back to an ancient Oriental proverb.

Chapter 6 - Script

In his book *Between Give and Take*, the Hungarian-American Ivan Boszormenyi Nagy writes intensely about the loyalty of children to the context and system from which they come. He points out, among other things, that – even though ties are broken – children continue to remain inextricably connected to their parents. A bit closer to home, but also exceptionally inspiring and inspired by TA, Piet Weisfelt has written about the significance of the family we are born into in his book *Nestgeuren*. He has inspired me to use the script circle he developed. Finally, for the diehards amongst us, I recommend *Lifescripts*; a hard to read, yet beautiful book edited by Richard Erskine, in which he reveals recent views on script development in relation to the development of our brain, the significance of the environment and the interplay between them.

Chapter 7 - Components of Script

Robert and Mary Goulding wrote a variety of books together, including the valuable book *Changing Lives Through Redecision* Therapy. In this book they describe how they work with injunctions and help people make re-decisions in and about their lives. With their method of working, the Gouldings created the redecision school of TA.

Mil Rosseau used the Goulding's work in his book with the amusing title: *Alleen natte baby's houden van verandering,* translated into English as: *Only wet babies like change.* In this book Rosseau applies the redecision concepts to the work situation. His book inspired me to use the road sign metaphor.

Taibi Kahler created the concept of drivers and incorporated it into the *process communication model*: www.kahlercommunications.com .

Sander Reinalda wrote an article titled: 'I want to be the Best'. This article can be downloaded from the Institute of Developmental Transactional Analysis website in the *IDTA Newsletter* that appeared in 2005 at http://www.instdta.org/idta-newsletters.html

Chapter 8 - Strokes

Claude Steiner, who I mentioned earlier, has written a lot about strokes in his life. In recent years his main focus has been on strokes within the context of the development of emotional intelligence. His books called *Achieving Emotional Literacy* and *The Heart of the Matter* are very worthwhile to read. He makes a distinction between emotional intelligence and emotional literacy: emotional intelligence with a heart.

Chapter 9 - Emotions

In his book *Bang boven boos* (translated into English as: *Fear above anger*), Henk Galenkamp writes about the effect of emotions on school safety. In this book, a flexible mind will be able to find sufficient basis to apply Galenkamp's thinking into other environments.

I found the chain diagram of racket feelings in the substantial book called *Passe-partout,* by Wibe Veenbaas. This book consists of many fundamental diagrams and theories from Transactional Analysis, Neuro-Linguistic Programming (NLP) and Systemic work and is, in my opinion, an indispensable reference book.

Chapter 10 - Working With Your Script Patterns

The redecision work within TA was created by Bob and Mary Goulding, as mentioned before. DVD's on which you can see the Gouldings at work are for sale via ITAA (International Transactional Analysis Association): www.itaa-net.org.

Rosemary Napper and Trudy Newton's book *Tactics* provides many tools for the development and learning of new behaviour. I have used a number of exercises from *Tactics* in this chapter and others. The chart that shows you how to work with your drivers is a modification of the chart that can be found in *Tactics*.

To conclude, I would like to mention that NLP has greatly influenced the way I look at development. The sentence 'behaviour you want to get rid of was the best choice you could ever have made' has always given me a lot of support. It has become an important guideline for how I look at and comprehend the behaviour of others as well as my own behaviour. There is a substantial amount of NLP literature on the market. Lucas Derks and Jaap Hollander wrote a valuable seminal book called *Essenties van NLP (Essence of NLP).*

Chapter 11 - Windows on The World

The life positions were initially described by Eric Berne, comprehensively covered in his book *What Do You Say After You Say Hello*, published in 1972. At a later stage, Franklyn Ernst developed the so-called *OK Corral* that he wrote about in his book *Who's Listening?* Subsequently, Julie Hay created the image of 'the windows on the world', an image that is probably more recognisable for Europeans. She describes 'the windows on the world' in her noteworthy book *Working it Out at Work* in which she converts TA models into terms that can be more easily understood, relating them specifically to what happens at work.

How life positions are perceived within TA has been greatly influenced by thinkers within the field of existential psychology and philosophy. Jean Paul Sartre wrote a lot about the relationship between 'me and the other', as did Viktor Frankl. The core focus of Martin Buber's work has been on 'I and Thou' as being inseparably linked to each other. I would also like to mention Levinas who (according to Duyndam & Poorthuis), like Buber, focussed mainly on 'the relation with the other' in his work. In contrast to Buber, he placed this in the context of 'the difference that exists between you and I'.

Chapter 12 - Transference

A lot has been written on transference in the history of psychotherapy. Distinction is made between transference (from client to therapist) and countertransference (from therapist to client). Petruska Clarkson gives a very clear description of these terms in her book *Transactional Analysis Psychotherapy: An Integrated Approach*.

Transference is key in the method created by the Relational school in TA that Helena Hargaden and Charlotte Sills write about in their book *Transactional Analysis, A Relational Perspective*. A difficult subject, but noteworthy for people who are interested in deepening their knowledge on this aspect of TA. Outside of the psychotherapeutic field, Fee van Delft describes the phenomenon of transference in layman's terms in her book *Overdracht en tegenoverdracht (Transference and countertransference)*.

Chapter 13 - Games

Eric Berne's *Games People Play*, written in 1967, unexpectedly became a bestseller. In an amusing way, Berne gives us insight into the games people play. The book is still available.

If you read this (or other TA books about games) note that Julie Hay suggested the changes to names of games given by Eric Berne: from NIGYSOB to Gotcha; from Wooden Leg to Millstone (i.e around my neck); and she always changes Rapo to Rebuff to avoid the connotation of rape being something 'invited' by the victim.

Menco Danen and Conny ten Klooster gave me permission to make use of their unissued article *'Over vastlopen en weer vlot trekken' (Run aground and getting afloat again)*. A download of their article is available via my website: www.lieuwe.net.

Petruska Clarkson developed the exceptionally valuable concept of 'the bystander', also the title of her book: *The Bystander*.

The Winner's Triangle was created by Acey Choy. The TA Journal published an article by Choy about this concept in 1990.

Chapter 14 - Symbiosis

The best book on this subject is Jacqui Lee Schiff's *Cathexis Reader*. This book is only available at an antiquarian bookseller, for instance via amazon.com. I have a very worn and faded copy on my bookshelf, filled with both my own and others' notes and scribbles.

The road map I used in this chapter was inspired by the *Cathexis Reader*, but actually borrowed and modified from Anne de Graaf and Klaas Kunst's book *Einstein en de kunst van het zeilen (Einstein and the art of sailing)*; a practical book about TA in the workplace, full of exercises, questionnaires and anecdotes. This book is avavailable in English from Sherwood Publishing in the UK www.sherwoodpublishing.com. Much of that book was in turn based on material by Julie Hay, whose books are available from the same publisher.

Chapter 15 - Vital Energy and Courage To Live

So far, the concept of Thymos hasn't been used in TA. However, I find that it combines very nicely with the term Physis. It helps me to understand why people aren't able to achieve their desires and what they need, so they will be able to do so. Thymos is an ancient Greek word. Plato writes about it in *The Republic*, in which he describes Thymos as the part of the soul that stands for passion and courage. Later philosophers, such as Thomas Aquinas, Spinoza and Kierkegaard, write about courage in various forms.

Paul Tillich wrote the inspiring book *The Courage to Be*, a splendid title although the splendour is not easy to discover because the book is hard to read. Recently, the German philosopher Peter Sloterdijk wrote about how necessary it is in these times that courageous people let go of old habits in order to create change in the world around us. In his essay *Rage and Time*, he too uses the word Thymos in relation to courage. Not long ago, Peter Venmans also wrote about the same theme in his noteworthy book *Het derde deel van de ziel (The third part of the soul)*.

About Transactional Analysis

Transactional Analysis (TA) is contemporaneous with and often regarded as part of humanistic psychology. TA is a theory of personality and it also provides us with a model of communication. TA's focus is on the ability of people to grow. Eric Berne founded TA in the 1950's and 1960's. Berne, an American, Canadian-born, psychiatrist, worked to become a psychoanalyst. However, he never completed his training. He gradually lost confidence in psychoanalysis and developed his own ideas and approach to psychotherapy.

Berne developed a goal-oriented therapy using simple images, models and metaphors in order to give patients greater power over their treatment and to help them take responsibility for their own development. At the time, Berne's thinking was very much in line with the societal developments in the 1960's and the existentialist thinking of philosophers such as Sartre and Camus.

Near to the end of his life, Berne also wrote about the use of Transactional Analysis within organisations.

In the 1960's he connected with a group of therapists who supported and further developed his ideas. Leading exponents of this group whose work has influenced me particularly include Claude Steiner, Fanita English and Thomas Harris. It was Harris who, at the beginning of the 1970's, wrote the worldwide bestseller *I'm OK, You're OK*.

In the 1970's TA was labelled as a 'pop-psychology': a popular version of psychology lacking in empirical evidence. Therefore TA gradually fell off the radar as a form of therapeutic aid, although many TA concepts were still being taught in trainings for psychologists, psychiatrists and medics. Since then it has become increasingly well-recognised as a therapeutic approach, with recognition via Masters degrees within several European countries.

TA had found its way to the fields of education, counselling, coaching and organisational consulting. There is now a masters for developmental TA applications (i.e. non-psychotherapy) of TA - see www.icdta.net. Currently, many people worldwide practice TA and they continue to develop TA. This has resulted and still gives rise to a steady stream of publications and, increasingly more, validated scientific research. Each quarter, an edition of the scientific *Transactional Analysis Journal* (TAJ) is issued. This journal publishes articles focussing on the four important fields of TA: psychotherapy, educational, organisational and counselling. In addition, there is the *International Journal of Transactional Analysis Research*, published twice a year, showcasing just how much research has been, and continues to be available to demonstrate the efficacy and effectiveness of TA. In 2018 this journal extended its coverage to include '*Practice*' across the variety of ways in which TA is applied internationally. The latter is available with free access for all at www.ijtarp.org.

Transactional Analysis has a well-defined certification system. The path leading to qualification in each of the four fields mentioned above, as well as certified membership of the European Association of Transactional Analysis (EATA) and/or the International Transactional Analysis Association (ITAA), consists of many hours of schooling, training and professional supervision. On average it takes about five to seven years to become a certified member.

Training in TA – whether for personal or professional growth – is offered around the world by institutes and certified individuals. To find out what training is available in your region, visit the website of the TA association nearest you. Those in the UK are the **UK Association for Transactional Analysis** (UKATA – formerly ITA), the **Institute of Developmental Transactional Analysis** (IDTA), the **Scottish Transactional Analysis Association** (STAA) and the **International Association for Relational Transactional Analysis** (IARTA). These professional bodies:

> promote, manage and sustain the application and growth of Transactional Analysis
> represent TA regionally, nationally and internationally
> establish and validate standards
> regulate and monitor ethical and professional practices of members
> act to advance the education of the public regarding the theory and practice of TA

The IDTA focuses on the non-psychotherapy applications of TA – the organisational, educational, counselling fields – which includes people working as consultants, trainers, educators, teachers, facilitators, counsellors, coach/mentors, HR professionals, etc. IDTA is a Partner Organisation with ITAA. Although based in the UK, IDTA has an international membership. See www.instdta.org. IDTA also operates a TA Proficiency Award scheme for teaching TA to children and to teachers, parents, caregivers and so on.

UKATA is a member of the UK Council for Psychotherapy, operates to UKCP criteria and standards for training, and is listed in the UKCP register as an accredited training agency. See http://www.uktransactionalanalysis.co.uk.

UKATA, IDTA, STAA (www.scottishta.org.uk) and IARTA (www.relationalta.com) are each affiliated to EATA (European Association of Transactional Analysis). Affiliation ensures that these bodies can represent the interests of UK members to the international community, participate in policy and decision making at all levels, and inform UK members of international developments. Membership of an affiliated body offers automatic membership of EATA.

Membership of these associations is open to anyone with an interest in TA. Different membership categories cater for those with a general interest, for people seeking professional training, and for those with international accreditation as Transactional Analysts.

The **International Transactional Analysis Association** (ITAA) offers direct membership in any area of the world. It also runs international conferences and publishes an academic journal and newsletter. See www.itaaworld.org.

The **International Centre for Developmental Transactional Analysis** operates various awards and qualifications, including an MSc accredited by a UK University, vocational awards for application of TA within various occupations, practitioner awards for those qualified in a non-TA approach, and advanced qualifications that can be credited towards the MSc and/or the international CTA qualification. See www.icdta.net.

Glossary of important concepts in Transactional Analysis

This glossary has been drafted with use of the *Dictionary of Transactional Analysis* by Tony Tilney and *TA Today: A New Introduction to Transactional Analysis.* (Second Edition) Ian Stewart & Vann Joines

Authentic feeling
A feeling that is felt spontaneously and without internal censoring and as such is congruent with experience. In TA four authentic feelings are distinguished: fear, anger, happiness and sadness.

Autonomy
Every behaviour, thought or feeling in response to here-and-now reality instead of them being controlled by script beliefs. Autonomy becomes apparent when a person (re)gains four capabilities: integrity, awareness, spontaneity and intimacy.

Awareness
The ability to experience emotional impressions purely, without immediately interpreting them.

Discounting
Unconsciously ignoring information that is relevant in order to solve a problem.

Drama Triangle
Diagram devised by Stephen Karpman on to which many patterns of interpersonal interaction can be mapped. It illustrates how people can take on three (script driven) positions or roles (Persecutor, Rescuer, Victim) and as the action unfolds the participants may move around the triangle and change roles. This movement around the triangle is characteristic of *games*.

At a later stage, Clarkson added the role of the bystander to the Drama Triangle. The Drama Triangle is mainly used to analyse *games*.

Drivers
Brief observable behaviours, which represent a defensive reaction to underlying *injunctions*. When a person is in driver they are dealing with internal stress arising from negative messages (injunctions) from early childhood.

Ego-state

A consistent pattern of feeling and experience directly related to a corresponding consistent pattern of behaviour. Three types of ego-states are distinguished in TA:

- Parent ego-state: the totality of behaviours, thoughts and feeling patterns taken from parents or parent figures experienced in the past, that is to say a 'borrowed' ego-state.
  Adult ego-state: the totality of behaviours, thoughts and feelings that are a direct response to the here-and-now.
  Child ego-state: the totality of feelings, behaviours and thoughts repeated from childhood.

Game

A process in which a person does something with an ulterior motive, which (1) occurs out of Adult awareness, (2) does not become explicit until participants suddenly switch their behaviour, and (3) results in each participant feeling confused and misunderstood whilst blaming the other for causing these feelings.

Grandiosity

An exaggeration of some aspect of reality often combined with discounting.

Injunctions

Negative, limiting script messages.

Integrating Adult

Adult ego-state in which all that is of value in the Child and Parent ego-state are integrated in the course of the life process.

Intimacy

A way of time structuring in which people communicate authentic feelings and needs to each other openly without censuring.

Life position

One's basic belief about oneself and others, used to justify one's decisions and behaviour.

Life script

An unconscious life plan derived from early experiences in childhood that governs the way life is lived out in a certain recurring sequence: experiences upheld (or confirmed?) by the parents, 'justified' by successive events, ending in an unconsciously pre-determined result.

Message at psychological level

A covert message, usually conveyed non verbally.

Message at social level

An open message, usually conveyed verbally.

Passive behaviour
One of the four forms of behaviour (doing nothing, over-adaption, agitation, incapacitation or violence), that is an indication of the occurrence of discounting. The individual uses either one of these forms of behaviour in an attempt to manipulate others or the social environment into solving his or her problem.

Permission
A message that something is allowable and OK. Permissions are positive and can liberate an individual from script messages.

Racket
A behaviour or sequence of behaviours that, out of awareness, is intended as a means to manipulate the social environment and that results in a racket feeling.

Racket feeling
A familiar, inauthentic feeling, learned and encouraged in childhood, which one experiences in stressful situations and is inadequate for problem resolution in a here-and-now manner.

Redecision
Replacement of an early self-limiting decision with a new decision using adult possibilities the individual has at his or her disposal.

Rubber band
A similarity between a stressful situation in the here-and-now and a painful childhood experience from a person's past they are usually unaware of. In reaction to this, the person will abruptly be inclined to move into their script.

Spontaneity
The ability to freely choose how to react from a broad range of options with regard to feeling, thinking and behaviour.

Stroke
A unit of recognition. TA distinguishes positive, negative, conditional and unconditional strokes. Strokes can be given either verbally or non-verbally.

Stroke economy
The set of parental rules with regard to giving and receiving strokes.

Stroke filter
An individual's pattern of either rejecting or accepting strokes, befitting their existing self-image.

Symbiosis
A relationship in which one or more individuals behave as though they constitute a single person. Neither of them are using their abilities.

Time structuring
People have a basic need for structure ('structure hunger'). This leads to the development of patterns or forms of time structuring, either alone, with another person or in a group.

Transaction
A transactional stimulus from one person to the other followed by a transactional response. The transaction is the unit of social intercourse.

Transactional Analysis
A theory of personality and a systematic psychotherapy for the benefit of personal growth and change.

References

References for authors mentioned in the book

Aquinas, Thomas – rather than choose a specific publication to reference, I suggest an internet search if you are not already familiar with this author

Barrow, Giles www.crackingbehaviour.com accessed 20 November 2016

Berne, Eric (1977) *Intuition and Ego States* New York: Harper & Row

Berne, Eric, (2010) *Games people play, the psychology of human relationships* Penguin Books Ltd.

Boszormenyi-Nagy, Ivan and Krasner, Barbara R. (1986) *Between Give and Take: A Clinical Guide To Contextual Therapy* Brunner/Mazel

Bowlby, John (1996) *Attachment and Loss, Volume 1 Attachment* Pimlico

Buber, Martin (1971) *I and Thou* New York: Charles Scribner's Sons

Camus, Albert (2000) *The Rebel* (trans Anthony Bower) London: Penguin Modern Classics - plus there are many others if you search the internet

Choy, Acey (1990) The Winner's Triangle *Transactional Analysis Journal* 20:1 40-46

Clarkson, Petruska (1992) *Transactional Analysis Psychotherapy: an Integrated Approach* Routledge

Clarkson, Petruska (1992) *The Bystander (an End to Innocence in Human Relations)* Whurr Publishers

Clarkson, Petruska (1992) Physis in Transactional Analysis *Transactional Analysis Journal* 22:4 202-209

De Graaf, Anne & Klaas Kunst (2005) *Einstein en de kunst van het zeilen, een zoektocht naar de nieuwe rol van de leidinggevende* Uitgeverij SWP. Published in English (2010) as *Einstein and the Art of Sailing: A New Perspective on the Role of Leadership* Hertford: Sherwood Publishing

Delft, Fee van (2004) *Overdracht en tegenoverdracht, een therapeutisch fenomeen vertaald naar alledaagse psychosociale begeleiding, Transference and countertransference, a therapeutic phenomenon translated to daily psycho-social work* Uitgeverij Nelissen

Derks, Lucas & Hollander, Jaap (1996) *Essenties van NLP* (Essences of NLP) Servire

Drego, Pearl A. (1993) Paradigms and Models of Ego States, *Transactional Analysis Journal* 23:1 5-29

Duyndam, Joachim en Poorthuis, Marcel (2005) *Levinas, serie Kopstukken in filosofie,* (Levinas, Leading Lights in Philosophy) Lemniscaat

English, Fanita (1971) The Substitution Factor; Rackets and Real Feelings Part 1 *Transactional Analysis Journal* 1:4 225-230
English, Fanita (1972) Rackets and Real Feelings Part 2 *Transactional Analysis Journal* 2:1 23-25
Ernst, Franklin H. (1968) *Who's listening* Adresso' Set Publications
Erskine, Richard G. (red.) (2010) *Life Scripts, a Transactional Analysis of Unconscious Patterns* Karnac Books

Fiddelaars-Jaspers, Riet (2011) *Met mijn ziel onder de arm* (With my soul under my arm) In de Wolken
Frankl, Viktor E. (1963) *Man's Search for Meaning. An Introduction to Logotherapy* Boston: Beacon Press

Galenkamp, Henk (2006) *Bang voor boos, de invloed van emoties op veiligheid in de School,* (Afraid of anger, the influence of emotions on safety in the school) CPS
Goulding, Mary and Goulding, Robert L. (1997) *Changing lives through Redecision Therapy* revised and updated edition, Grove Press

Harris, Thomas A. (1967) *I'm OK – You're OK* Harper & Row
Hay, Julie (2009) *Working It Out At Work. Understanding Attitudes and Building Relationships (2nd Edition)* Sherwood Publishing

James, Muriel M. (1973) *Born to love, Transactional Analysis in the Church* Addison Wesley
James, Muriel and James, John (1992) *Passion for life* Plume
Jung, Carl Gustav (2002) *Answer to Job* Routledge Classic

Kahler, Taibi www.kahlercommunications.com accessed 20 November 2016
Kierkegaard, Søren – rather than choose a specific publication to reference, I suggest an internet search if you are not already familiar with this author
Klooster, Conny ten en Danen, *Menco Over vastlopen en weer vlot trekken', interne publicatie voor leerlingenbegeleiding HvA.* (about crashing and getting on the road again) Internal publication HvA
Kohlrieser, George (2006) *Hostage at the table* Jossey Bass
Koopmans, Lieuwe (2010) Functional Fluency *Strook* June

Levin, Pamela (1998) *Cycles of Power, a User's Guide to the Seven Seasons of Life* Health Communications
Levin, Pamela (1988) *Becoming the Way We Are* Health Communications
Lips, Roek (2011) *Ben ik in beeld?,* (Am I on The Spot?) FC Klap

Napper, Rosemary and Newton, Trudy (2003) *Tactics* TA-resources
Nietzche, Friedrich (1991) *The Gay Science* (trans Walter Kaufman) Mass Market Paperback

Parr, John *The Feeling Wheel: a Tool for Systematic Analysis of Feelings* MSc Thesis, a non-published article, used with prior consent.

Plato (1995) *Constitutie Politeia* Athenaeum-Polak 7 Van Gennep

Reinalda, Sander (2005) I want to be the best *IDTA Newsletter* 2: 6 6-8

Rosseau, Mil (2007) *Alleen natte baby's houden van verandering: versnellen van persoonlijke ontwikkeling en verandering in organisaties,* (Only wet babies like to change) Acco

Sartre, Jean Paul (2007) *Existentialism and Humanism* York: Methuen Books – plus there are many others if you search the internet

Schiff, Jacqui Lee & Contributors (1975) *Cathexis Reader, Transactional Analysis Treatment of Psychosis* Harper & Row

Sills, Charlotte and Hargaden, Helena (eds) (2002) *Ego States* Worth Publishing

Sills, Charlotte and Hargaden Helena (2002) *Transactional Analysis, a Relational Perspective* Routledge

Sloterdijk, Peter (2010) *Rage and Time* Columbia University Press

Spinoza,Benedict – rather than choose a specific publication to reference, I suggest an internet search if you are not already familiar with this author

Steiner, Claude M. (1971) The Stroke Economy *Transactional Analysis Journal* 1:3 9-15

Steiner, Claude M. (2003) *Emotional Literacy, Intelligence with a Heart* Personhood Press

Steiner, Claude M. (2009) *The Heart of the Matter* TA-Press

Steiner, Claude www.claudesteiner.com

Stewart, Ian and Joines, Vann (2012) *TA Today, a New Introduction to Transactional Analysis* (second edition), Lifespace Publishing

Temple, Susannah (1999) Functional Fluency for Educational Transactional Analysts *Transactional Analysis Journal* 29:3 164-174

Temple, Susannah (2004) Update on the Functional Fluency Model in Education *Transactional Analysis Journal* 34:3 197-204

Temple, Susannah www.functionalfluency.com

Tillich, Paul (2000) *The Courage to be* Yale University Press

Tilney, Tony (1998) *Dictionary of Transactional Analysis* Whurr Publishers

Tudor, Keith (2003) The Neopsyche: the Integrating Adult ego state in C. Sills & H Hargaden (eds) *Ego States*. London: Worth Publishing 201-231

Veenbaas, Wibe E A (2007) *Passe Partout* (Master Key) Phoenix Opleidingen

Veenbaas, Wibe and Goudswaard Joke (2002) *Vonken van verlangen, systemisch werk, perspectief en praktijk,* (Sparkles of Longing, Systemic work perspective and practice) Phoenix Opleidingen

Venmans, Peter (2011) *Het derde deel van de ziel* (The third part of the soul) Uitgeverij Atlas

Viorst Judith (2003) *Necessary Losses* Prentice Hall

Weisfelt, Piet (1996) *Nestgeuren en de betekenis van de ouder-kindrelatie in een mensenleven,* (The smell of the nest and the meaning of parent-child relationship in life) Uitgeverij Nelissen

References for other publications that have inspired me

Bor, Jan, (2010) *Een (nieuwe) geschiedenis van de filosofie,* (A (new) history of philosophy) Uitgeverij Bert Bakker

Cialdini, Robert B. (2000) *Influence, Science and Practice* 4th edition Allyn & Bacon
Cornell, William F. (1988) Life Script Theory; a Critical Review from a Developmental Perspective *Transactional Analysis Journal* 18:4 270-282

Iacoboni, Marco (2009) Imitation, Empathy, and Mirror Neurons *Annual Review of Psychology* 60: 653-670

Widdowson, Mark (2010) *Transactional Analysis, 100 Key Points & Techniques* Routledge

Made in the USA
Monee, IL
07 July 2026

56553286R00079